NUTRITION AND DIET RESEARCH PROGRESS

PROTEIN DIETS

NUTRITIONAL SOURCES, HEALTH BENEFITS AND INTAKE RECOMMENDATIONS

NUTRITION AND DIET RESEARCH PROGRESS

Additional books in this series can be found on Nova's website under the Series tab.

Additional e-books in this series can be found on Nova's website under the e-book tab.

NUTRITION AND DIET RESEARCH PROGRESS

PROTEIN DIETS

NUTRITIONAL SOURCES, HEALTH BENEFITS AND INTAKE RECOMMENDATIONS

MEAGHAN HUDSON
EDITOR

nova publishers
New York

Library of Congress Cataloging-in-Publication Data

ISBN: 978-1-63463-498-4

Library of Congress Control Number: 2014955177

Published by Nova Science Publishers, Inc. † New York

CONTENTS

PREFACE

Protein is an essential macronutrient in the human diet. In addition to providing essential amino acids to the body, protein has also been linked to inducing the feeling of fullness and satiety. Different sources of protein are traditionally used in the human diet and offer varying amino acid composition. This book discusses the nutritional sources of protein, as well as its health benefits and intake recommendations.

Chapter 1 - The proportion of US adults over the age 65 and the prevalence of obesity in older adults have increased dramatically. The incidence of obesity in older adults has coincided with an increase in the progression and development of cardiometabolic and skeletal muscle dysfunction, which may be further exacerbated by age-related muscle loss (i.e., sarcopenic obesity). Dietary interventions that effectively induce weight loss and attenuate cardiometabolic and skeletal muscle loss are clearly warranted, although there is concern that excessive weight loss may accelerate age-related muscle and bone loss. Several studies have demonstrated that weight loss induced by energy restriction, physical activity, or a combination of both, when coupled with an increase in dietary protein intake at levels above the US recommended dietary allowance (RDA: 0.8 $g \cdot kg^{-1} \cdot d^{-1}$) may be an effective strategy that promotes healthy weight loss. More specifically, consuming a high protein (1-1.5 $g \cdot kg^{-1} \cdot d^{-1}$), moderate carbohydrate diet (~40% total energy intake) promotes the loss of body fat and attenuates the loss of lean body mass induced by weight loss. Emerging evidence also suggests that equal distribution of high quality, high protein meals throughout the day enhances 24-h muscle protein synthesis, which may offset age-related anabolic resistance to dietary protein and contribute to the maintenance of lean body mass. High protein, weight loss diets may also increase intestinal calcium absorption which may result in long-term preservation in bone mineralization. Increasing dietary protein at the expense of carbohydrate may also improve dyslipidemia, enhance insulin sensitivity, and upregulate hepatic gluconeogenesis during weight loss. This chapter will review the implications of obesity in older adults on cardiometabolic and skeletal muscle status, with emphasis on sarcopenic obesity. Potential metabolic benefits of high protein, moderate carbohydrate weight loss diets will be discussed, and the mechanisms by which dietary protein confers metabolic protection will be explored.

Chapter 2 - Hepatic encephalopathy (HE) is a spectrum of neuropsychiatric abnormalities in patients with chronic liver disease. Since the late nineteenth century, protein restriction has been shown to improve hepatic encephalopathy. However, malnutrition has been well documented in a large proportion of cirrhotic patients and it has been shown to be associated with increased mortality. Emerging clinical evidence has revealed that a large proportion of cirrhotic patients with HE tolerate normal protein intake without aggravation of their underlying encephalopathy. Nonetheless, in approximately one-third of patients on maximal medical therapy are documented to be protein-sensitive. In this selected group of patients, modifying their sources for nitrogen with use of vegetable-based proteins and branched-chain amino acids may be necessary to improve their encephalopathy without further loss of lean body mass. Current evidence shows that protein supplementation does not necessarily exacerbate HE in a majority of cirrhotic patients and can improve outcome. In patients with severe HE, short-term protein restriction or modification of dietary protein sources should be considered in cases of HE that are refractory to maximal medical therapy.

Chapter 3 - Protein is an essential macronutrient in the human diet. In addition to providing essential amino acids to the body, protein has also been linked to inducing the feeling of fullness and satiety. Different sources of protein are traditionally used in the human diet and offer varying amino acid composition. This chapter will summarize work on the implications of the amount and type of protein in the diet to promote the control of hunger and fullness (satiety). Furthermore, evidence regarding the short-term implications of high protein diets on colonic microbiota, fermentation and ultimately intestinal health is presented.

Chapter 4 - Structurally, proteins are macromolecules composed of basic amino acid units linked by peptide bonds (amino group of an amino acid bound to the carboxyl group of another amino acid). In terms of nutrition, what distinguishes one protein from another is its amino acid intake. There are 22 amino acids that form proteins, however, only 10 of them are considered nutritionally essential, which are among the nutrients that more impact animal performance.Therefore, it is of fundamental importance to know the food's amino acid composition, as well as its use by animals. Among the protein sources, soybean meal is an ingredient widely used in feed due to its balance of amino acids, on the other hand, like other plant foods, it has anti-nutritional factors that can affect the absorption and utilization of nutrients, especially in young animals.Animal byproducts can also be a good protein alternative with high digestibility, palatability and free of anti-nutritional factors.

Protein digestion begins in the stomach, where pepsin cleaves some peptide bonds. Like many other enzymes related to the digestion of proteins, pepsins are secreted as inactive precursors (proenzymes) and are activated in the gastrointestinal tube. The precursors of pepsin are called pepsinogen and are activated by gastric hydrochloric acid.

In poultry, food does not remain long in the proventriculus, passing quickly tothe ventriculus. At this stage of the digestive process the contractions of the wall grind the food, increasing its contact surface with the enzymes. However as well as in mammals, the protein digestion to polypeptides depends on factors such as the residence time of food in the proventriculus and the physical characteristic of the ingested protein.

To provide an adequate utilization of proteins from food, the first step is the degradation in the gastrointestinal tract (GIT) to the level of amino acids and small peptic chains so that absorption occurs.In order for this to happen, animals have a number of enzymes present in the digestive fluids which act in many different ways. Understanding this mechanism of digestion and enzyme activity in proteins in the GIT is important for defining protein digestibility of foods and therefore the biological value of protein.

The interest in researching appropriate protein recommendations for poultry and pigs has grown over the years due to factors such as increased protein sources' prices thus raising feed costs, greater availability of affordable industrial amino acid and limitation of nitrogen excretion predicted by environmental legislation.

Previously, diets for animals were formulated based on crude protein. In this concept, the amino acid amount was provided in excess or unbalanced resulting in nitrogen loss. Thus, the ideal protein concept emerged, which is to provide without excess or deficiency the amount of amino acids needed to meet the requirements for maintenance and production of the animal.

The ideal protein concept makes the diet economic by reducing waste of the second nutrient that most raises feed costs. Moreover it also prevents the additional energy expense to excrete amino acid that is supplied in excess, since it is not used by the animals as a source of protein. Finally, this prevents eliminated nutrient is released into the environment causing negative environmental pollution impact.

The ideal protein concept allows a decrease in protein levels provided once the proper level of limiting amino acids is maintained with industrial amino acids' supplementation in order not to impair the animal's performance. However, this requires formulating diets based on true digestible amino acids considering the relationship that exists between them, with lysine as reference.

Amino acids can be classified as essential, conditionally essential, and nonessential. Essential amino acids are those that animals can't produce a significant amount; conditionally essential are those that are, in a given situation, produced in insufficient quantities; and not essential are produced efficiently by animals. Essential amino acids are lysine, methionine, threonine, tryptophan, valine, leucine, isoleucine, phenylalanine, histidine and tyrosine.

The amino acids requirements for poultry and swine may vary due to several factors, such as nutrient levels, the animal's age, genetics and gender. Thus, many studies have been conducted to estimate protein and amino acid requirement considering these factors. Therefore, this chapter analyzes the main requirement recommendations of protein and amino acids for poultry and swine cited in the literature, as Rostagno et al., (2011), NRC (2012) and scientific papers published in leading scientific journals.

In this paper, sources, recommendation and protein metabolism in poultry and swine are discussed.

In: Protein Diets
Editor: Meaghan Hudson

ISBN: 978-1-63463-498-4

Chapter 1

EFFECTS OF DIETARY PROTEIN ON METABOLIC HEALTH IN OBESE OLDER ADULTS

Lee M. Margolis, Holly L. McClung and Stefan M. Pasiakos

Military Nutrition Division, US Army Research Institute of Environmental Medicine, Natick, MA, US

ABSTRACT

The proportion of US adults over the age 65 and the prevalence of obesity in older adults have increased dramatically. The incidence of obesity in older adults has coincided with an increase in the progression and development of cardiometabolic and skeletal muscle dysfunction, which may be further exacerbated by age-related muscle loss (i.e., sarcopenic obesity). Dietary interventions that effectively induce weight loss and attenuate cardiometabolic and skeletal muscle loss are clearly warranted, although there is concern that excessive weight loss may accelerate age-related muscle and bone loss. Several studies have demonstrated that weight loss induced by energy restriction, physical activity, or a combination of both, when coupled with an increase in dietary protein intake at levels above the US recommended dietary allowance (RDA: 0.8 $g \cdot kg^{-1} \cdot d^{-1}$) may be an effective strategy that promotes healthy weight loss. More specifically, consuming a high protein (1-1.5 $g \cdot kg^{-1} \cdot d^{-1}$), moderate carbohydrate diet (~40% total energy intake) promotes the loss of body fat and attenuates the loss of lean body mass induced by weight loss. Emerging evidence also suggests that equal distribution of high quality, high protein meals throughout the day enhances 24-h muscle protein synthesis, which may offset age-related anabolic resistance to dietary protein and contribute to the maintenance of lean body mass. High protein, weight loss diets may also increase intestinal calcium absorption which may result in long-term preservation in bone mineralization. Increasing dietary protein at the expense of carbohydrate may also improve dyslipidemia, enhance insulin sensitivity, and upregulate hepatic gluconeogenesis during weight loss. This chapter will review the implications of obesity in older adults on cardiometabolic and skeletal muscle status, with emphasis on sarcopenic obesity. Potential metabolic benefits of high protein, moderate carbohydrate weight loss diets will be discussed, and the mechanisms by which dietary protein confers metabolic protection will be explored.

INTRODUCTION

The proportion of the US population over 65 years old is greater now than ever before [1] and is projected to continue to grow over the next several decades [2]. Compromised musculoskeletal mass is a consistent pathophysiological change with aging, due to age-related decrements in skeletal muscle mass (sarcopenia) [3] and bone mineralization (osteoporosis) [4]. These degenerative processes can impair locomotion, mobility, and physical function [5]. The decline in physical activity and loss of metabolically active peripheral tissue generally occurs with concomitant decrements in resting energy expenditure [6], resulting in the accumulation of body fat (sarcopenic obesity) [7]. Changes in body composition can further exacerbate sarcopenia, as gains in body fat occur with progressive declines in skeletal muscle mass [8, 9]. Furthermore, the increase in body fat increases the accumulation of triglycerides in hepatic tissue and skeletal muscle, which typically alters glucose homeostasis and blood lipids [10, 11].

Although energy restriction induces favorable changes in total body mass, fat mass, metabolic and cardiovascular risk [12, 13], weight loss strategies have been highly contentious for older adults [14] as they may exacerbate age-related declines in muscle mass [15] and bone mineralization [16, 17].

However, there is increasing evidence to suggest that increasing dietary protein intake to levels approaching twice the recommended dietary allowance (RDA) is an effective nutritional approach to spare muscle mass and promote the loss of body fat [18-22], without compromising bone mineralization during weight loss [23]. Furthermore, increased protein intake at the expense of carbohydrate may also enhance glycemic regulation and reduce atherogenic dyslipidemia [24, 25]. High carbohydrate diets have been shown to be atherogenic, and they upregulate *de novo* lipogenesis, and induce hypertriglyceridemia [26, 27]. Elevated triglyceride concentrations result in further accumulation of hepatic and intramuscular triglycerides resulting in diminished cardiometabolic health [28]. This chapter will review the effects of obesity in older adults on skeletal muscle and bone mineralization, and explore potential health-related benefits of high protein diets for older adults.

Dietary Protein and Maintenance of Skeletal Muscle Mass during Weight Loss

Dietary protein is a primary regulator of skeletal muscle mass modulating muscle protein turnover, and particularly the upregulation of muscle protein synthesis (MPS) [29]. Dietary protein stimulates MPS through amino acid-induced signaling of the mammalian target of rapamycin complex 1 (mTORC1) [30, 31]. In the postabsorptive state, net protein balance is negative, as MPS rates are generally lower than muscle protein breakdown (MPB). Under non-diseased conditions, MPB is upregulated during fasting to liberate endogenous amino acids which sustain blood glucose and energy production [32]. Consuming a protein-containing meal stimulates MPS and attenuates MPB, resulting in a net anabolic state that persists for approximately 2 hours before returning to postabsorptive levels [33, 34]. The overall balance between MPS and MPB determines whether an individual gains, maintains, or loses muscle mass over time [35].

Weight loss and aging alter muscle protein turnover [36, 37], which in turn contributes to skeletal muscle mass loss [36, 38]. Weight loss is inherently catabolic, with intentional negative energy balance induced to stimulate reductions in total mass and fat mass. However, with these desired losses, there is an unintentional loss of skeletal muscle mass [15]. Reductions in skeletal muscle mass are due to increased metabolic demand for amino acids as substrates for hepatic gluconeogenesis [39]. These alterations in protein metabolism may blunt postprandial MPS in response to a protein-containing meal [18]. While the cause of age-associated losses in muscle mass is multifactorial, postprandial MPS is blunted with aging, which alters protein requirements to achieve optimal anabolic responses to feeding [40-42].

Increasing the total amount and optimizing the distribution of dietary protein intake throughout the day may be effective strategies to improve protein balance and reduce the loss of skeletal muscle in older adults attempting weight loss [43, 44]. Protein intake equaling twice the RDA spares muscle and increases the loss of body fat during weight loss [18-22]. Maintenance of postabsorptive and postprandial MPS may account for the benefit of protein on muscle mass with weight loss [45]. Consuming higher amounts of protein attenuated energy deficit-induced decrements in postprandial MPS [18, 46], which likely contributed to the preservation of muscle mass [18]. The distribution and timing of a high protein diet may be equally as important as the total amount of protein consumed during weight loss. Maximal stimulation of MPS in response to dietary protein appears to be saturated at approximately 0.25-0.3 g/kg per meal (~18-23 g protein per meal for an average 75 kg [165 lb] male), suggesting that both level and timing should be considered when trying to optimize dietary responses to weight loss [47]. Studies have demonstrated that 20 g of an isolated, high-quality protein or 30 g of protein within a mixed-meal maximally stimulates MPS [34, 40, 48, 49]. Consuming protein in excess of these amounts increases protein oxidation with no further increase in MPS [50], perhaps contributing nothing more than increased energy intake. As many adults skew their protein intake, with low levels of protein consumed at breakfast (< 15 g) and high levels consumed at dinner (> 30 g) [51], they are likely not optimizing MPS. Eating in a pattern when there is equal distribution of protein at each meal may promote a more sustained MPS response over the course of the day [52, 53], as Mamerow et al. [54] reported that MPS over 24 hours was 25% higher when protein intake was distributed evenly between meals (breakfast: ~30 g, lunch: ~30 g, dinner: ~30 g) compared to a more traditional skewed protein intake (breakfast: ~11 g, lunch: ~16 g, dinner: ~63 g). As such, equal distribution of a high protein diet throughout the day is likely muscle protective during weight loss.

Relationship of Dietary Protein and Bone Health

Reductions in bone mineralization are unavoidable with aging [4]. When considered in light of the age-related muscle loss, which increases the risk of falls, there is a greater risk of fracture, and frailty. The overall compromise of the musculoskeletal system may worsen sarcopenic obesity [55].

There is a growing body of evidence that suggests increased protein intake may be protective and mitigate bone loss [56], as consuming protein at levels consistent with the RDA may exacerbate bone loss [57]. Historically, high protein diets were believed to compromise bone health by increasing calcium excretion [58]. The prevailing hypothesis was that increased calcium excretion was due to mobilization of calcium from bone to buffer the increased acid load produced by protein catabolism [59, 60], resulting in a reduction in bone mineral density and progression of osteoporosis [59]. Evidence now shows that dietary protein may impart benefit, or, at a minimum, may not be detrimental to bone. Studies using stable isotope methodologies to assess calcium absorption and retention have reported that increased calcium excretion induced by high protein diets is a result of a concomitant increase in intestinal calcium absorption [61, 62]. These findings indicate that high protein-induced calcium excretion is a result of increased intestinal calcium absorption, not a result of bone demineralization. Weight loss may exacerbate bone demineralization [16, 17]. However, several studies have reported that high protein weight loss diets with adequate calcium intake attenuate losses in bone mineral density [63-65]. Cao et al. [66] recently demonstrated that following 21 days of moderate weight loss (negative energy balance 1000 $kcal \cdot d^{-1}$), there was no difference in calcium retention or biomarkers of bone turnover when comparing protein intakes equivalent to the RDA, twice the RDA or three times the RDA. This further supports the theory that dietary protein above the RDA will not compromise bone health.

Influence of Dietary Protein on Glycemic Control and Cardiovascular Health

The prevalence of obesity in older adults has increased the progression of cardiometabolic-related comorbidities [67]. Obesity reflects increased fat deposition in the form of triglycerides in subcutaneous and visceral adipose tissue, and, to an extent, skeletal muscle [68].

Increased intramuscular triglycerides (IMTG) may alter metabolic processes, specifically glycemic regulation [69] and insulin sensitivity [70-72] (Figure 1). The progression of obesity-induced insulin resistance appears to be mediated through protein kinase θ (PKC θ). PKC θ inhibits the activation of insulin receptor substrates (IRS), which under normal physiological conditions stimulates downstream intracellular signaling and translocation of glucose transport 4 (GLUT4) in response to insulin by phosphorylating AKT substrate of 160 kDa (AS160) [73].

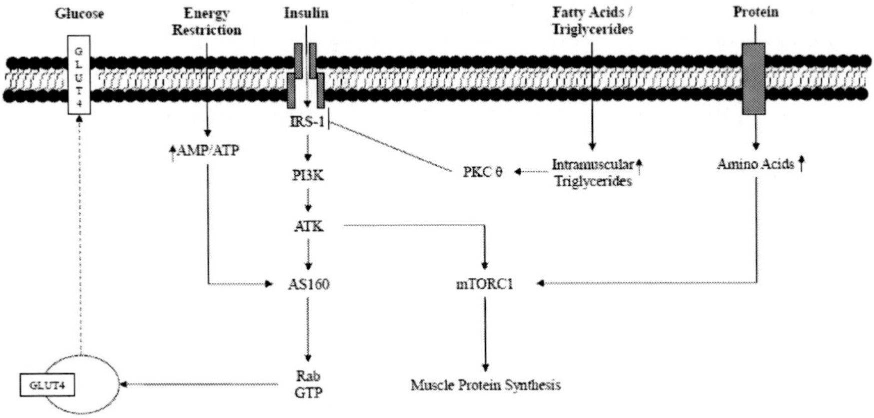

IRS; Insulin Receptor Substrate, PI3K; Phosphoinositide 3-Kinase, PKC θ; Protein Kinase C θ, AS160; AKT substrate of 160 kDa, GTP; Guanosine-5'-triphosphate, mTORC1; mammalian Target of Rapamycin Complex 1, GLUT4; Glucose Transporter 4.

Figure 1. Intracellular signaling regulation of GLUT4 translocation and activation of mTORC1. Elevated intramuscular triglycerides reduce insulin sensitivity, diminishing translocation of GLUT4 to the cellular membrane for glucose uptake. Insulin stimulates mTORC1 through AKT, increased intramuscular triglycerides may diminish muscle protein synthesis.

Inhibition of GLUT4 translocation reduces skeletal muscle glucose uptake and subsequent glucose oxidation and glycogen synthesis, thereby promoting hyperglycemia.

The alteration in insulin sensitivity and increased accumulation of IMTG accompanying obesity may also negatively impact MPS, partially accounting for the observed anabolic resistance with aging and progression of sarcopenia in obese older adults. Reduced insulin-mediated MPS [74-76] is likely due to an inhibition of AKT, a downstream target of IRS, which when phosphorylated stimulates the activation of mTORC1.

While amino acids initiate activation of mTORC1 independent of AKT, increased IMTG impede the sensitivity of MPS to dietary protein intake [76].

This impaired response to feeding has been attributed to lipid accumulation in skeletal muscle resulting in activation of localized proinflammatory cytokines, tumor necrosis factor alpha (TNFα) and nuclear factor kappa-light-chain enhancer of activated B cells (NFκB) [77, 78].

Increased IMTG levels may also downregulate mTORC1 activity [79], and upregulate activation lipogenic regulators fatty acid synthase (FAS), and acetyl CoA carboxylase (ACC) [80, 81].

Weight loss alone can reduce fat stores and improve insulin sensitivity and insulin-mediated glucose uptake through activation of AMP-activated protein kinase (AMPK). AMPK phosphorylates AS160 to stimulate GLUT4 translocation [82] and decrease IMTG [83]. Further improvements in glycemic control and diminished IMTG may be achieved with high protein, low carbohydrate weight loss diets. High carbohydrate diets have been shown to potentiate adverse health outcomes with obesity through persistent elevation of glucose levels and *de novo* lipogenesis [84]. Excess intracellular glucose from carbohydrate intake beyond what is required for energy metabolism and glycogen storage will stimulate *de novo* lipogenesis through the conversion of Acetyl CoA to Malonyl CoA [84] (Figure 2). The practice of altering carbohydrate intake by increasing protein consumption during weight loss has been shown to improve glycemic control and decrease triglyceride concentrations [25]. Lower carbohydrate intake generally results in lower postprandial blood glucose, insulin secretion [22, 85], and *de novo* lipogenesis [25, 86]. Diminished glucose availability increases reliance on exogenous protein and fatty acids to maintain energy and glucose production. Lipolysis is upregulated during weight loss, as fatty acids become the primary endogenous substrate for gluconeogenesis and energy production [87].

Elevated protein intake at the expense of carbohydrate appears to enhance these adaptions to energy deficit, resulting in greater reductions in intracellular markers of lipogenesis, including Acetyl-CoA Carboxylase (ACC) and Fatty Acid Synthase (FAS), and increased markers of hepatic [88] and skeletal muscle gluconeogenesis (PEPCK) [89].

Improved glycemic control and reduced IMTG resulting from high protein diets also improves insulin sensitivity [90, 91], β-cell function [91], and diminishes glycated hemoglobin percentage (HbA1c) [85]. Improved insulin sensitivity and decrements in body fat resulting from high protein, weight loss diets may also be cardiometabolic protective, as insulin resistance contributes to the progression of dyslipidemia and atherosclerosis [92]. Specifically, increased protein intake has been consistently reported to diminish circulating triglycerides during weight loss, often to a greater extent than high carbohydrate diets [20, 25, 93]. Furthermore, while weight loss alone improves lipoprotein profiles by reducing total and low density lipoprotein (LDL) cholesterol levels, high protein, weight loss diets may also increase high density lipoprotein (HDL) cholesterol [94, 95]. Thus, comparing high protein (1-1.5 $g \cdot kg^{-1} \cdot d^{-1}$) to high carbohydrate (55-60 % of total energy intake), weight loss diets, high protein diets elicit a lower triglyceride-to-HDL and LDL-to-HDL ratio, which is indicative of a lower risk for cardiometabolic disease [96].

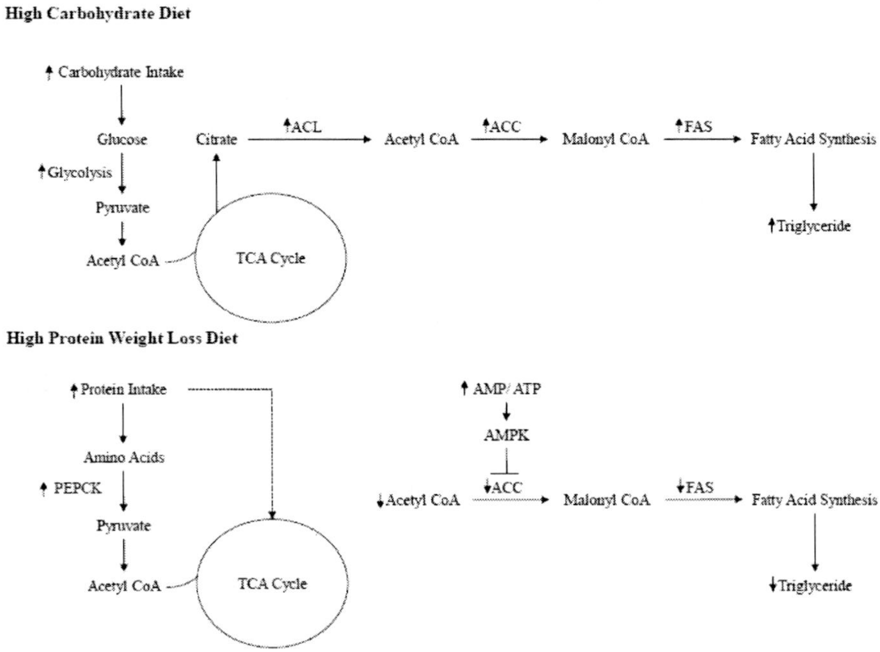

ACL; ATP Citrate Lyase, ACC; Acetyl CoA Carboxylase, FAS; Fatty Acid Synthase, PEPCK; Phosphoenolpyruvate Carboxykinase, AMPK; AMP Activated Protein Kinase.

Figure 2. Excess carbohydrate intake beyond the amount required for energy production and glycogen storage is synthesized into fatty acids through the conversion of Acetyl CoA to Malonyl CoA via ACC. High protein weight loss diets increase amino acid-derived energy production and reduce Acetyl CoA accumulation. Activity of ACC is also blunted by the upregulation of AMPK with energy restriction, resulting in diminished fatty acid synthesis.

Conclusion

It is clear that increasing dietary protein intake to levels approaching twice the RDA is an effective nutritional strategy for sparing skeletal muscle and bone mineralization in obese older adults during weight loss. The distribution of dietary protein in meals may be equally as important as the total amount of protein in the diet, although this hypothesis has not been tested in the context of weight loss and lean body mass. High protein, low carbohydrate weight loss diets also appear to be an effective strategy to manage cardiometabolic status by enhancing glycemic control and lipid profiles.

The opinions or assertions contained herein are the private views of the authors and are not to be construed as official or as reflecting the views of the Army or the Department of Defense. Any citations of commercial organizations and trade names in this report do not constitute an official Department of the Army endorsement of approval of the products or services of these organizations.

REFERENCES

[1] *Federal Integagency Forum On Aging-Related Statistics.* Older Americans 2012: Key Indicators of Well-Being. 2012; 2-10.

[2] Administration on Aging. *A Profile of Older Americans:* 2012. 2012; 1-4.

[3] Evans, W. J., Campbell, W. W. Sarcopenia and age-related changes in body composition and functional capacity. *J. Nutr.*, 1993;123(2 Suppl.): 465-8.

[4] Exton-Smith, A. N., Millard, P. H., Payne, P. R., Wheeler, E. F. Pattern of development and loss of bone with age. *Lancet*, 1969;2(7631):1154-7.

[5] Fielding, R. A., Vellas, B., Evans, W. J., Bhasin, S., Morley, J. E., Newman, A. B., Abellan van Kan, G., Andrieu, S., Bauer, J., Breuille, D., Cederholm, T., Chandler, J., De Meynard, C., Donini, L., Harris, T., Kannt, A., Keime Guibert, F., Onder, G., Papanicolaou, D., Rolland, Y., Rooks, D., Sieber, C., Souhami, E., Verlaan, S., Zamboni, M. Sarcopenia: an undiagnosed condition in older adults. Current consensus definition: prevalence, etiology, and consequences. International working group on sarcopenia. *J. Am. Med. Dir. Assoc.*, 2011;12(4): 249-56.

[6] Manini, T. M. Energy expenditure and aging. *Ageing Res. Rev.* 2010;9 (1):1-11.

[7] Stenholm, S., Harris, T. B., Rantanen, T., Visser, M., Kritchevsky, S. B., Ferrucci, L. Sarcopenic obesity: definition, cause and consequences. *Curr. Opin. Clin. Nutr. Metab. Care*, 2008;11(6):693-700.

[8] Parr, E. B., Coffey, V. G., Hawley, J. A. 'Sarcobesity': a metabolic conundrum. *Maturitas*, 2013;74(2):109-13.

[9] Baumgartner, R. N., Wayne, S. J., Waters, D. L., Janssen, I., Gallagher, D., Morley, J. E. Sarcopenic obesity predicts instrumental activities of daily living disability in the elderly. *Obes. Res.*, 2004;12(12):1995-2004.

[10] Kelley, D. E., Goodpaster, B. H. Skeletal muscle triglyceride. An aspect of regional adiposity and insulin resistance. *Diabetes Care*, 2001;24 (5): 933-41.

[11] Galbo, T., Shulman, G. I. Lipid-induced hepatic insulin resistance. *Aging*, 2013;5(8):582-3.

[12] Blackburn, G. Effect of degree of weight loss on health benefits. *Obesity research* 1995;3 Suppl. 2:211s-6s.

[13] Pasanisi, F., Contaldo, F., de Simone, G., Mancini, M. Benefits of sustained moderate weight loss in obesity. *Nutr. Metab. Cardiovasc. Dis.*, 2001;11(6):401-6.

[14] Waters, D. L., Ward, A. L., Villareal, D. T. Weight loss in obese adults 65years and older: a review of the controversy. *Exp. Gerontol.*, 2013;48 (10):1054-61.

[15] Weinheimer, E. M., Sands, L. P., Campbell, W. W. A systematic review of the separate and combined effects of energy restriction and exercise on fat-free mass in middle-aged and older adults: implications for sarcopenic obesity. *Nutr. Rev.*, 2010;68(7):375-88.

[16] Shapses, S. A., Riedt, C. S. Bone, body weight, and weight reduction: what are the concerns? *J. Nutr.*, 2006;136(6):1453-6.

[17] Pritchard, J. E., Nowson, C. A., Wark, J. D. Bone loss accompanying diet-induced or exercise-induced weight loss: a randomised controlled study. *Int. J. Obes. Relat. Metab. Disord.*, 1996;20(6):513-20.

[18] Pasiakos, S. M., Cao, J. J., Margolis, L. M., Sauter, E. R., Whigham, L. D., McClung, J. P., Rood, J. C., Carbone, J. W., Combs, G. F., Jr, Young, A. J. Effects of high-protein diets on fat-free mass and muscle protein synthesis following weight loss: a randomized controlled trial. *FASEB J.,* 2013;27(9):3837-47.

[19] Mettler, S., Mitchell, N., Tipton, K. D. Increased protein intake reduces lean body mass loss during weight loss in athletes. *Med. Sci. Sports Exerc.*, 2010;42(2):326-37.

[20] Layman, D. K., Boileau, R. A., Erickson, D. J., Painter, J. E., Shiue, H., Sather, C., Christou, D. D. A reduced ratio of dietary carbohydrate to protein improves body composition and blood lipid profiles during weight loss in adult women. *J. Nutr.*, 2003;133(2):411-7.

[21] Gordon, M. M., Bopp, M. J., Easter, L., Miller, G. D., Lyles, M. F., Houston, D. K., Nicklas, B. J., Kritchevsky, S. B. Effects of dietary protein on the composition of weight loss in post-menopausal women. *J. Nutr. Health Aging,* 2008;12(8):505-9.

[22] Farnsworth, E., Luscombe, N. D., Noakes, M., Wittert, G., Argyiou, E., Clifton, P. M. Effect of a high-protein, energy-restricted diet on body composition, glycemic control, and lipid concentrations in overweight and obese hyperinsulinemic men and women. *Am. J. Clin. Nutr.*, 2003; 78(1):31-9.

[23] Tang, M., O'Connor, L. E., Campbell, W. W. Diet-induced weight loss: the effect of dietary protein on bone. *J. Acad. Nutr. Diet.*, 2014;114 (1): 72-85.

[24] Layman, D. K., Evans, E. M., Erickson, D., Seyler, J., Weber, J., Bagshaw, D., Griel, A., Psota, T., Kris-Etherton, P. A moderate-protein diet produces sustained weight loss and long-term changes in body composition and blood lipids in obese adults. *J. Nutr.*, 2009;139(3):514-21.

[25] Layman, D. K., Clifton, P., Gannon, M. C., Krauss, R. M., Nuttall, F. Q. Protein in optimal health: heart disease and type 2 diabetes. *Am. J. Clin. Nutr.* 2008;87(5):1571S-5S.

[26] Parks, E. J., Hellerstein, M. K. Carbohydrate-induced hypertriacylglycerolemia: historical perspective and review of biological mechanisms. *Am. J. Clin. Nutr.*, 2000;71(2):412-33.

[27] McDevitt, R. M., Bott, S. J., Harding, M., Coward, W. A., Bluck, L. J., Prentice, A. M. De novo lipogenesis during controlled overfeeding with sucrose or glucose in lean and obese women. *Am. J. Clin. Nutr.*, 2001; 74(6):737-46.

[28] Kraegen, E. W., Cooney, G. J., Ye, J., Thompson, A. L. Triglycerides, fatty acids and insulin resistance--hyperinsulinemia. *Exp. Clin. Endocrinol. Diabetes*, 2001;109(4):S516-26.

[29] Wolfe, R. R. Regulation of muscle protein by amino acids. *J. Nutr.*, 2002;132(10):3219S-24S.

[30] Proud, C. G. Amino acids and mTOR signalling in anabolic function. *Biochem. Soc. Trans.,* 2007;35(Pt 5):1187-90.

[31] Drummond, M. J., Dreyer, H. C., Fry, C. S., Glynn, E. L., Rasmussen, B. B. Nutritional and contractile regulation of human skeletal muscle protein synthesis and mTORC1 signaling. *J. Appl. Physiol.*, 2009;106 (4):1374-84.

[32] Veldhorst, M. A., Westerterp-Plantenga, M. S., Westerterp, K. R. Gluconeogenesis and energy expenditure after a high-protein, carbohydrate-free diet. *Am. J. Clin. Nutr.*, 2009;90(3):519-26.

[33] Atherton, P. J., Etheridge, T., Watt, P. W., Wilkinson, D., Selby, A., Rankin, D., Smith, K., Rennie, M. J. Muscle full effect after oral protein:

time-dependent concordance and discordance between human muscle protein synthesis and mTORC1 signaling. *Am. J. Clin. Nutr.*, 2010;92 (5):1080-8.

[34] Bohe, J., Low, A., Wolfe, R. R., Rennie, M. J. Human muscle protein synthesis is modulated by extracellular, not intramuscular amino acid availability: a dose-response study. *J. Physiol.*, 2003;552(Pt 1):315-24.

[35] Tipton, K. D., Borsheim, E., Wolf, S. E., Sanford, A. P., Wolfe, R. R. Acute response of net muscle protein balance reflects 24-h balance after exercise and amino acid ingestion. *Am. J. Physiol. Endocrinol. Metab.*, 2003;284(1):E76-89.

[36] Breen, L., Phillips, S. M. Skeletal muscle protein metabolism in the elderly: Interventions to counteract the 'anabolic resistance' of ageing. *Nutr. Metab.*, 2011;8:68.

[37] Carbone, J. W., McClung, J. P., Pasiakos, S. M. Skeletal muscle responses to negative energy balance: effects of dietary protein. *Adv. Nutr.*, 2012;3(2):119-26.

[38] Pasiakos, S. M., Vislocky, L. M., Carbone, J. W., Altieri, N., Konopelski, K., Freake, H. C., Anderson, J. M., Ferrando, A. A., Wolfe, R. R., Rodriguez, N. R. Acute energy deprivation affects skeletal muscle protein synthesis and associated intracellular signaling proteins in physically active adults. *J. Nutr.*, 2010;140(4):745-51.

[39] Knapik, J., Meredith, C., Jones, B., Fielding, R., Young, V., Evans, W. Leucine metabolism during fasting and exercise. *J. Appl. Physiol.*, 1991; 70(1):43-7.

[40] Cuthbertson, D., Smith, K., Babraj, J., Leese, G., Waddell, T., Atherton, P., Wackerhage, H., Taylor, P. M., Rennie, M. J. Anabolic signaling deficits underlie amino acid resistance of wasting, aging muscle. *FASEB J.,* 2005;19(3):422-4.

[41] Katsanos, C. S., Kobayashi, H., Sheffield-Moore, M., Aarsland, A., Wolfe, R. R. Aging is associated with diminished accretion of muscle proteins after the ingestion of a small bolus of essential amino acids. *Am. J. Clin. Nutr.*, 2005;82(5):1065-73.

[42] Volpi, E., Rasmussen, B. B. Nutrition and muscle protein metabolism in the elderly. *Diabetes Nutr. Metab.*, 2000;13(2):99-107.

[43] Bauer, J., Biolo, G., Cederholm, T., Cesari, M., Cruz-Jentoft, A. J., Morley, J. E., Phillips, S., Sieber, C., Stehle, P., Teta, D., Visvanathan, R., Volpi, E., Boirie, Y. Evidence-based recommendations for optimal dietary protein intake in older people: a position paper from the PROT-AGE Study Group. *J. Am. Med. Dir. Assoc.*, 2013;14(8):542-59.

[44] Wycherley, T. P., Moran, L. J., Clifton, P. M., Noakes, M., Brinkworth, G. D. Effects of energy-restricted high-protein, low-fat compared with standard-protein, low-fat diets: a meta-analysis of randomized controlled trials. *Am. J. Clin. Nutr.*, 2012;96(6):1281-98.

[45] Phillips, S. M. Higher protein during an energy deficit: muscle's guardian and fat's enemy? *Medicine and science in sports and exercise* 2008;40(3):503-4.

[46] Areta, J. L., Burke, L. M., Camera, D. M., West, D. W., Crawshay, S., Moore, D. R., Stellingwerff, T., Phillips, S. M., Hawley, J. A., Coffey, V. G. Reduced resting skeletal muscle protein synthesis is rescued by resistance exercise and protein ingestion following short-term energy deficit. *Am. J. Physiol. Endocrinol. Metab.*, 2014;306(8):E989-97.

[47] Rodriguez, N. R. Protein-centric meals for optimal protein utilization: can it be that simple? *J. Nutr.*, 2014;144(6):797-8.

[48] Robinson, M. J., Burd, N. A., Breen, L., Rerecich, T., Yang, Y., Hector, A. J., Baker, S. K., Phillips, S. M. Dose-dependent responses of myofibrillar protein synthesis with beef ingestion are enhanced with resistance exercise in middle-aged men. *Appl. Physiol. Nutr. Metabol.*, 2013;38(2):120-5.

[49] Symons, T. B., Sheffield-Moore, M., Wolfe, R. R., Paddon-Jones, D. A moderate serving of high-quality protein maximally stimulates skeletal muscle protein synthesis in young and elderly subjects. *J. Am. Diet. Assoc.*, 2009;109(9):1582-6.

[50] Moore, D. R., Robinson, M. J., Fry, J. L., Tang, J. E., Glover, E. I., Wilkinson, S. B., Prior, T., Tarnopolsky, M. A., Phillips, S. M. Ingested protein dose response of muscle and albumin protein synthesis after resistance exercise in young men. *Am. J. Clin. Nutr.*, 2009;89(1):161-8.

[51] Service. UAR. Energy intakes: percentages of energy from protein, carbohydrate, fat, and alcohol, by gender and age, what we eat in America, NHANES 2009-2010. 2012, Avialable from: wwwarsusdagov/ba/bhnrc/fsrg.

[52] Layman, D. K. Dietary Guidelines should reflect new understandings about adult protein needs. *Nutr. Metab.*, 2009;6:12.

[53] Paddon-Jones, D., Rasmussen, B. B. Dietary protein recommendations and the prevention of sarcopenia. *Curr. Opin. Clin. Nutr. Metab. Care.* 2009;12(1):86-90.

[54] Mamerow, M. M., Mettler, J. A., English, K. L., Casperson, S. L., Arentson-Lantz, E., Sheffield-Moore, M., Layman, D. K., Paddon-Jones,

D. Dietary Protein Distribution Positively Influences 24-h Muscle Protein Synthesis in Healthy Adults. *J. Nutr.* 2014;144(6):876-80.

[55] Strasser, B. Physical activity in obesity and metabolic syndrome. *Ann. N Y Acad. Sci.,* 2013;1281:141-59.

[56] Dawson-Hughes, B. Calcium and protein in bone health. *Proc. Nutr. Soc.* 2003;62(2):505-9.

[57] Gaffney-Stomberg, E., Insogna, K. L., Rodriguez, N. R., Kerstetter, J. E. Increasing dietary protein requirements in elderly people for optimal muscle and bone health. *J. Am. Geriatr. Soc.* 2009;57(6):1073-9.

[58] Barzel, U. S., Massey, L. K. Excess dietary protein can adversely affect bone. *J. Nutr.*, 1998;128(6):1051-3.

[59] Jesudason, D., Clifton, P. The interaction between dietary protein and bone health. *J. Bone Miner. Metab.*, 2011;29(1):1-14.

[60] Heaney, R. P., Layman, D. K. Amount and type of protein influences bone health. *Am. J. Clin. Nutr.*, 2008;87(5):1567S-70S.

[61] Kerstetter, J. E., O'Brien, K. O., Caseria, D. M., Wall, D. E., Insogna, K. L. The impact of dietary protein on calcium absorption and kinetic measures of bone turnover in women. *J. Clin. Endocrinol. Metab.*, 2005; 90(1):26-31.

[62] Hunt, J. R., Johnson, L. K., Fariba Roughead, Z. K. Dietary protein and calcium interact to influence calcium retention: a controlled feeding study. *Am. J. Clin. Nutr.*, 2009;89(5):1357-65.

[63] Thorpe, M. P., Jacobson, E. H., Layman, D. K., He, X., Kris-Etherton, P. M., Evans, E. M. A diet high in protein, dairy, and calcium attenuates bone loss over twelve months of weight loss and maintenance relative to a conventional high-carbohydrate diet in adults. *J. Nutr.*, 2008;138(6): 1096-100.

[64] Bowen, J., Noakes, M., Clifton, P. M. A high dairy protein, high-calcium diet minimizes bone turnover in overweight adults during weight loss. *J. Nutr.*, 2004;134(3):568-73.

[65] Skov, A. R., Haulrik, N., Toubro, S., Molgaard, C., Astrup, A. Effect of protein intake on bone mineralization during weight loss: a 6-month trial. *Obes. Res.*, 2002;10(6):432-8.

[66] Cao, J. J., Pasiakos, S. M., Margolis, L. M., Sauter, E. R., Whigham, L. D., McClung, J. P., Young, A. J., Combs, G. F., Jr. Calcium homeostasis and bone metabolic responses to high-protein diets during energy deficit in healthy young adults: a randomized controlled trial. *Am. J. Clin. Nutr.,* 2014;99(2):400-7.

[67] Poirier, P., Giles, T. D., Bray, G. A., Hong, Y., Stern, J. S., Pi-Sunyer, F. X., Eckel, R. H., American Heart A, Obesity Committee of the Council on Nutrition PA, Metabolism. Obesity and cardiovascular disease: pathophysiology, evaluation, and effect of weight loss: an update of the 1997 American Heart Association Scientific Statement on Obesity and Heart Disease from the Obesity Committee of the Council on Nutrition, Physical Activity, and Metabolism. *Circulation*, 2006;113(6):898-918.

[68] Van Loon, L. J., Koopman, R., Manders, R., van der Weegen, W., van Kranenburg, G. P., Keizer, H. A. Intramyocellular lipid content in type 2 diabetes patients compared with overweight sedentary men and highly trained endurance athletes. *Am. J. Physiol. Endocrinol. Metab.*, 2004; 287(3):E558-65.

[69] Shulman, G. I. Cellular mechanisms of insulin resistance. *J. Clin. Invest.*, 2000;106(2):171-6.

[70] Roden, M., Price, T. B., Perseghin, G., Petersen, K. F., Rothman, D. L., Cline, G. W., Shulman, G. I. Mechanism of free fatty acid-induced insulin resistance in humans. *J. Clin. Invest.*, 1996;97(12):2859-65.

[71] Dresner, A., Laurent, D., Marcucci, M., Griffin, M. E., Dufour, S., Cline, G. W., Slezak, L. A., Andersen, D. K., Hundal, R. S., Rothman, D. L., Petersen, K. F., Shulman, G. I. Effects of free fatty acids on glucose transport and IRS-1-associated phosphatidylinositol 3-kinase activity. *J. Clin. Invest.*, 1999;103(2):253-9.

[72] Griffin, M. E., Marcucci, M. J., Cline, G. W., Bell, K., Barucci, N., Lee, D., Goodyear, L. J., Kraegen, E. W., White, M. F., Shulman, G. I. Free fatty acid-induced insulin resistance is associated with activation of protein kinase C theta and alterations in the insulin signaling cascade. *Diabetes*, 1999;48(6):1270-4.

[73] Szendroedi, J., Yoshimura, T., Phielix, E., Koliaki, C., Marcucci, M., Zhang, D., Jelenik, T., Muller, J., Herder, C., Nowotny, P., Shulman, G. I., Roden, M. Role of diacylglycerol activation of PKCtheta in lipid-induced muscle insulin resistance in humans. *Proc. Natl. Acad. Sci. US*, 2014;111(26):9597-602.

[74] Rasmussen, B. B., Fujita, S., Wolfe, R. R., Mittendorfer, B., Roy, M., Rowe, V. L., Volpi, E. Insulin resistance of muscle protein metabolism in aging. *FASEB J.,* 2006;20(6):768-9.

[75] Guillet, C., Prod'homme, M., Balage, M., Gachon, P., Giraudet, C., Morin, L., Grizard, J., Boirie, Y. Impaired anabolic response of muscle protein synthesis is associated with S6K1 dysregulation in elderly humans. *FASEB J.,* 2004;18(13):1586-7.

[76] Guillet, C., Delcourt, I., Rance, M., Giraudet, C., Walrand, S., Bedu, M., Duche, P., Boirie, Y. Changes in basal and insulin and amino acid response of whole body and skeletal muscle proteins in obese men. *J. Clin. Endocrinol. Metab.,* 2009;94(8):3044-50.

[77] Holland, W. L., Bikman, B. T., Wang, L. P., Yuguang, G., Sargent, K. M., Bulchand, S., Knotts, T. A., Shui, G., Clegg, D. J., Wenk, M. R., Pagliassotti, M. J., Scherer, P. E., Summers, S. A. Lipid-induced insulin resistance mediated by the proinflammatory receptor TLR4 requires saturated fatty acid-induced ceramide biosynthesis in mice. *J. Clin. Invest.,* 2011;121(5):1858-70.

[78] Giresi, P. G., Stevenson, E. J., Theilhaber, J., Koncarevic, A., Parkington, J., Fielding, R. A., Kandarian, SC. Identification of a molecular signature of sarcopenia. *Physiol. Genomics*, 2005;21(2):253-63.

[79] Chale-Rush, A., Morris, E. P., Kendall, T. L., Brooks, N. E., Fielding, R. A. Effects of chronic overload on muscle hypertrophy and mTOR signaling in young adult and aged rats. *J. Gerontol. A Biol. Sci. Med. Sci.*, 2009;64(12):1232-9.

[80] Haran, P. H., Rivas, D. A., Fielding, R. A. Role and potential mechanisms of anabolic resistance in sarcopenia. *J. Cachexia Sarcopenia Muscle,* 2012;3(3):157-62.

[81] Rivas, D. A., Morris, E. P., Fielding, R. A. Lipogenic regulators are elevated with age and chronic overload in rat skeletal muscle. *Acta Physiol.,* 2011;202(4):691-701.

[82] Treebak, J. T., Glund, S., Deshmukh, A., Klein, D. K., Long, Y. C., Jensen, T. E., Jorgensen, S. B., Viollet, B., Andersson, L., Neumann, D., Wallimann, T., Richter, E. A., Chibalin, A. V., Zierath, J. R., Wojtaszewski, J. F. AMPK-mediated AS160 phosphorylation in skeletal muscle is dependent on AMPK catalytic and regulatory subunits. *Diabetes*, 2006;55(7):2051-8.

[83] Houmard, J. A., Tanner, C. J., Yu, C., Cunningham, P. G., Pories, W. J., MacDonald, K. G., Shulman, G. I. Effect of weight loss on insulin sensitivity and intramuscular long-chain fatty acyl-CoAs in morbidly obese subjects. *Diabetes*, 2002;51(10):2959-63.

[84] Menezes, A. L., Pereira, M. P., Buzelle, S. L., Dos Santos, M. P., de Franca, S. A., Baviera, A. M., Andrade, C. M., Garofalo, M. A., Kettelhut Ido, C., Chaves, V. E., Kawashita, N. H. A low-protein, high-carbohydrate diet increases de novo fatty acid synthesis from glycerol

and glycerokinase content in the liver of growing rats. *Nutr. Res.*, 2013; 33(6):494-502.

[85] Gannon, M. C., Nuttall, F. Q., Saeed, A., Jordan, K., Hoover, H. An increase in dietary protein improves the blood glucose response in persons with type 2 diabetes. *Am. J. Clin. Nutr.*, 2003;78(4):734-41.

[86] Larsen, T. M., Dalskov, S. M., van Baak, M., Jebb, S. A., Papadaki, A., Pfeiffer, A. F., Martinez, J. A., Handjieva-Darlenska, T., Kunesova, M., Pihlsgard, M., Stender, S., Holst, C., Saris, W. H., Astrup, A., Diet, Obesity, and Genes (Diogenes) Project. Diets with high or low protein content and glycemic index for weight-loss maintenance. *N. Engl. J. Med.,* 2010;363(22):2102-13.

[87] Canto, C., Auwerx, J. Calorie restriction: is AMPK a key sensor and effector? *Physiol.* 2011;26(4):214-24.

[88] Freudenberg, A.,Petzke, K. J., Klaus, S. Comparison of high-protein diets and leucine supplementation in the prevention of metabolic syndrome and related disorders in mice. *J. Nutr. Biochem.*, 2012;23(11): 1524-30.

[89] Stepien, M., Gaudichon, C., Fromentin, G., Even, P., Tome, D., Azzout-Marniche, D. Increasing protein at the expense of carbohydrate in the diet down-regulates glucose utilization as glucose sparing effect in rats. *PloS one* 2011;6(2):e14664.

[90] Kim, H. H., Kim, Y. J., Lee, S. Y., Jeong, D. W., Lee, J. G., Yi, Y. H., Cho, Y. H., Choi, E. J., Kim, H. J. Interactive effects of an isocaloric high-protein diet and resistance exercise on body composition, ghrelin, and metabolic and hormonal parameters in untrained young men: A randomized clinical trial. *J. Diabetes Investig.*, 2014;5(2):242-7.

[91] Kitabchi, A. E., McDaniel, K. A., Wan, J. Y., Tylavsky, F. A., Jacovino, C. A., Sands, C. W., Nyenwe, E. A., Stentz, F. B. Effects of high-protein versus high-carbohydrate diets on markers of beta-cell function, oxidative stress, lipid peroxidation, proinflammatory cytokines, and adipokines in obese, premenopausal women without diabetes: a randomized controlled trial. *Diabetes Care*, 2013;36(7):1919-25.

[92] Grundy, S. M. Small LDL, atherogenic dyslipidemia, and the metabolic syndrome. *Circulation*, 1997;95(1):1-4.

[93] Skov, A. R., Toubro, S., Ronn, B., Holm, L., Astrup, A. Randomized trial on protein vs carbohydrate in ad libitum fat reduced diet for the treatment of obesity. *Int. J. Obes. Relat. Metab. Disord.*, 1999;23(5): 528-36.

[94] Parker, B., Noakes, M., Luscombe, N., Clifton, P. Effect of a high-protein, high-monounsaturated fat weight loss diet on glycemic control and lipid levels in type 2 diabetes. *Diabetes Care*, 2002;25(3):425-30.

[95] Krauss, R. M., Blanche, P. J., Rawlings, R. S., Fernstrom, H. S., Williams, P. T. Separate effects of reduced carbohydrate intake and weight loss on atherogenic dyslipidemia. *Am. J. Clin. Nutr.* 2006;83(5): 1025-31.

[96] Penalva, R. A., Huoya Mde, O., Correia, L. C., Feitosa, G. S., Ladeia, A. M. Lipid profile and intensity of atherosclerosis disease in acute coronary syndrome. *Arq. Bras. Cardiol.*, 2008;90(1):24-30.

In: Protein Diets
Editor: Meaghan Hudson

ISBN: 978-1-63463-498-4

Chapter 2

MODIFICATION OF PROTEIN INTAKE MAY BE NECESSARY IN SELECTED PATIENTS WITH HEPATIC ENCEPHALOPATHY

Matthew A. Chin, M.D.[1], Matthew L. Bechtold M.D.[2], and Douglas L. Nguyen, M.D.[1*]

[1]University of California, Irvine Division of Gastroenterology and Hepatology, US
[2]University of Missouri, Columbia Division of Gastroenterology and Hepatology, MO, US

ABSTRACT

Hepatic encephalopathy (HE) is a spectrum of neuropsychiatric abnormalities in patients with chronic liver disease. Since the late nineteenth century, protein restriction has been shown to improve hepatic encephalopathy. However, malnutrition has been well documented in a large proportion of cirrhotic patients and it has been shown to be associated with increased mortality. Emerging clinical evidence has revealed that a large proportion of cirrhotic patients with HE tolerate normal protein intake without aggravation of their underlying encephalopathy. Nonetheless, in approximately one-third of patients on

* Corresponding Author: Douglas Nguyen, M.D., Assistant Clinical Professor of Medicine, Division of Gastroenterology and Hepatology, 101 The City Drive, Orange, CA 92697, (714) 456-6745, douglaln@uci.edu.

maximal medical therapy are documented to be protein-sensitive. In this selected group of patients, modifying their sources for nitrogen with use of vegetable-based proteins and branched-chain amino acids may be necessary to improve their encephalopathy without further loss of lean body mass. Current evidence shows that protein supplementation does not necessarily exacerbate HE in a majority of cirrhotic patients and can improve outcome. In patients with severe HE, short-term protein restriction or modification of dietary protein sources should be considered in cases of HE that are refractory to maximal medical therapy.

INTRODUCTION

Hepatic encephalopathy, or porto-systemic encephalopathy, represents a spectrum of neuropsychiatric disease in patients with liver disease, ranging from subtle changes in behavior only detectable by psychometric testing, to confusion, to altered level of consciousness and coma. The development of encephalopathy in patients with chronic liver disease is a sign of decompensation, and may be indicative of a poor prognosis. Important factors contributing to the development of hepatic encephalopathy include degree of hepatic failure, portosystemic shunting, and exogenous factors such as infection and variceal bleeding [1].

While the syndrome of hepatic encephalopathy reflects a complex interchange between reversible metabolic encephalopathy, brain atrophy and edema, and neurotransmitter derangement, the main tenant in its pathogenesis centers around the concept that nitrogenous substances derived from the gut adversely affect brain function. Ammonia, gamma-aminobutyric acid-ergic (GABA-ergic), catecholamine pathways, and other false neurotransmitters have been implicated. In patients with hepatic encephalopathy, therapy is based around addressing the underlying causes and undertaking strategies to reduce intake, production, and absorption of such neurotoxic substances.

MALNUTRITION IN CHRONIC LIVER DISEASE

Protein calorie malnutrition has been reported in up to 60% of patients with decompensated liver disease [2]. Several population studies have consistently demonstrated that malnutrition is a significant contributor to morbidity and mortality of patients with chronic liver disease [3,4]. Furthermore, malnutrition among cirrhotic patients has been associated with variceal bleeding, refractory ascites, spontaneous bacterial peritonitis, and hepatorenal syndrome [5-7].

Despite its prevalence and clinical significance, malnutrition in chronic liver disease remains under diagnosed and undermanaged due to its complex pathogenesis [8]. In a recent single-center European study, up to 60% of physicians underestimated their patients' nutritional requirements, and, as a consequence, recommended lower energy intakes than considered adequate [9]. The lack of reliable biomarkers that accurately reflect the nutritional status of patients with cirrhosis can complicate this question.

Decreased nutritional intake is driven by means of chronic nausea and abdominal discomfort from ascites, and malabsorption by means of altered bile salt metabolism, impaired digestion, and bowel edema [10]. Patients with cirrhosis suffer metabolic derangements through insulin resistance, impaired glycogen storage, and increased basal metabolic rate [11-13]. Finally, iatrogenic insults including prolonged periods of limited oral intake during frequent hospitalizations and drug or toxin-induced malnutrition may play a role.

Protein Intake and Hepatic Encephalopathy

For more than half a century, protein restriction has one of the mainstay treatments for hepatic encephalopathy [14-17]. The goal of a low-protein dietary strategy is to reduce intestinal ammonia production, which is implicated as a key factor in the pathogenesis of hepatic encephalopathy [18-20]. Because skeletal muscle tissue plays a crucial role in removing circulating ammonia, loss of this "ammonia sink" in the malnourished patient may play a role in driving encephalopathy [21, 22]. Clinical observation has shown that high protein intake may worsen encephalopathy in approximately 35% of cirrhotic patients [1]. The dilemma for clinicians rests in the managing a delicate balance of nutrition and encephalopathy.

In 2004 Cordoba et al. published the first prospective, randomized controlled study of cirrhotics with hepatic encephalopathy who received different amounts of dietary protein [23]. Of 62 patients considered for the study, 30 were ultimately enrolled, with 15 receiving 1.2 g/kg/day, and 15 initially receiving no protein, then, after 3 days, having their intake increased slowly to 1.2 g/kg/day. Exclusionary criteria included acute alcoholic hepatitis, GI bleeding, and terminal illness. In all patients, the primary cause of hepatic encephalopathy was treated, and patients were also given lactulose and neomycin. At the time of study conclusion at 14 days, protein synthesis and degredation, biochemical data (including ammonia), and the clinical course of encephalopathy were all similar in the two groups.

The Cordoba study was not without limitations. Randomization may have been inadequate; for example, the average baseline weight was 60kg in the low-protein group and 69kg in the normal-protein group. Only 20 patients were analyzed and nearly one-third of enrolled patients died. The type of dietary protein administered was not classified in the study. Therefore, while it may be reasonable to conclude that selected patients with acute hepatic encephalopathy who are on maximum medical therapy may tolerate nutritional support with 1.2 g/kg/day of protein, the study may not be able to be uniformly applied to all cirrhotic patients. Notably, the Cordoba study also demonstrated that short-term protein restriction may not result in significant total body protein turnover. In cases of medically refractory hepatic encephalopathy, there may still be a role for the safe administration of short-term protein restriction, as observed in historical cohorts.

While many cirrhotic patients can tolerate a high protein diet without induction or exacerbation of hepatic encephalopathy, it is recognized that a subset of patients are protein-intolerant [24]. Gheorghe at al. demonstrated in a series of 122 patients with hepatic encephalopathy that 80% were able to tolerate a high-calorie, high casein-vegetable protein diet without further deterioration of mental status [25]. Of those patients who required a brief course of protein restriction, clinical improvement in encephalopathy was observed for nearly 70%.

Modification of Dietary Nitrogen Sources

Sources of Proteins

The 2001 American College of Gastroenterology Practice Guidelines on Hepatic Encephalopathy provide the recommendation that for cirrhotic patients with acute encephalopathy, protein intake should be started at 0.5 g/kg/day with subsequent progressive increase to 1.0-1.5 g/kg/day, depending on patient tolerance, [26] however, the European Society for Parenteral and Enteral Nutrition (ESPEN) guidelines, updated in 2006 (after the Cordoba study), recommend that all patients with cirrhosis should have a goal protein intake of at least 1.2 g/kg/day [27].

However, the type of protein consumed may be as important as the total amount of protein ingested, as patients have different tolerance of dietary protein. Early historical studies have shown that dairy protein may be better tolerated than protein from mixed sources, and vegetable protein may be better tolerated than meat [28-31].

One benefit from a diet higher in vegetable protein is the higher intake of dietary fiber than isonitrogenous meat protein diets, which increases intestinal food transit, increased fecal ammonia excretion, and reduction in colonic lumen pH, which prevents gut ammonia absorption and may result in a more favorable fecal mictrobiota [32-34].

Meat-based protein is higher than vegetable protein in sulfated amino acids methionine and cysteine, which are precursors to mercaptans and indole and/or oxindole compounds which have been implicated in the pathogenesis of hepatic encephalopathy [35]. By contrast, vegetable proteins are high in ornithine and arginine, which help facilitate ammonia disposal through the urea cycle [36].

In studies that provided a head-to-head comparison of vegetable protein and meat protein diets, results have consistently favored the former. In a study of patients with mild chronic hepatic encephalopathy, Uribe et al. demonstrated improvement in mental state, number connection test times and electroencephalograms in those given a vegetable protein diet compared to those on animal protein diets plus neomycin [37]. In a second study by Bianchi et al. patients with chronic encephalopathy despite lactulose therapy who were given seven days of a vegetable protein diet had improvement in nitrogen balance, serum ammonia, and clinical grading and psychometric testing, while those on a meat protein diet did not [38].

A 2011 consensus statement by the International Society for Hepatic Encephalopathy and Nitrogen Metabolism recommends that patients with recurrent hepatic encephalopathy eat a diet low in animal protein in favor for one rich in vegetable protein; consistent with the 2006 ESPEN guidelines which favor vegetable protein once encephalopathy has developed [20,27]. It is worth noting, however, that more than 30-40 g of vegetable protein per day may cause significant diarrhea and abdominal bloating, after which time, it may be reasonable to supplement with dairy products to increase a patient's protein intake [39]. It is important to recognize that, despite minimization or avoidance of meat protein for patients with hepatic encephalopathy, a subset of patients might still benefit from a brief period of protein restriction [25].

Branched Chain Amino Acids

The branched-chain amino acids (BCAAs) valine, leucine, and isoleucine are essential amino acids which are metabolized in skeletal muscle and play a role in gluconeogenesis, and protein synthesis, and are catabolized into glutamine, which acts as a substrate for ammonia detoxification [40]. It has been demonstrated that levels of serum BCAAs are reduced in patients with cirrhosis, while aromatic amino acids (AAAs), are increased [41]. This imbalance may result in increased passage of AAAs across the blood brain barrier, where they are metabolized into false neurotransmitters that drive encephalopathy [42]. BCAAs can be administered orally or intravenously and for the past few decades their role in patients with hepatic encephalopathy has been a subject of close study.

Their success has been demonstrated by a large multicenter study from Italy, in which significant improvement in psychometric testing was appreciated in patients with chronic hepatic encephalopathy who were given BCAAs [43]. A Cochrane review of 11 randomized-controlled trials, comprising of 556 patients with hepatic encephalopathy demonstrated a statistically significant improvement in patients administered BCAAs, with encephalopathy improving in 59% in the BCAA groups at the end of treatment verses 41% of controls (RR 1.31, 95% CI 1.04-1.66) [44]. However, the analysis failed to demonstrate an effect on time to improvement or overall survival. Additionally, many of the included studies had significant limitations; studied populations were small (ranged from 22-75 patients), with short follow up periods, (6-30 days, 7 of the 11 studies did not report their follow up range). When only high quality studies were included, the benefit of BCAAs on hepatic encephalopathy was extinguished.

There have been several large quality studies that do suggest a limited role for the use of BCAAs. In a randomized, multicenter trial of 646 patients with decompensated cirrhosis and a study period of two years, patients given BCAAs experienced reduction in a composite end point of death, hepatocellular carcinoma, rupture of esophageal varices, and progression of hepatic failure, in addition to improved levels of serum albumin and improved patient self-assessment of overall health [45]. In a second randomized, multicenter trial of 174 patients and a study period of 1 year, the use of BCAAs resulted in a reduced rate of hospital admission, improvement in Child-Pugh score, and quality of life, although long-term compliance was poor and there was no difference in encephalopathy [46]. In a recent randomized controlled trial of 116 patients with cirrhosis, BCAAs failed to prevent recurrent hepatic encephalopathy, but did result in improvement in muscle mass [47].

The 2006 ESPEN guidelines suggest that there may be a role for BCAAs in medically refractory hepatic encephalopathy [27]. In a subset of patients who are protein-intolerant, reducing protein intake and supplementing with BCAAs may maintain lean body mass without aggravating hepatic encephalopathy. However, their routine use remains limited by the lack of evidence of improved overall mortality, poor availability, high costs, and limited patient compliance.

Conclusion

Malnutrition remains a common condition among cirrhotic patients, and is a harbinger of an increased risk for complications such as variceal bleeding, refractory ascites, spontaneous bacterial peritonitis, and hepatorenal syndrome.

Historically, protein restriction has been shown to improve hepatic encephalopathy, however, emerging evidence suggests that a large portion of cirrhotic patients may be able to tolerate a normal level of protein intake. In the subset of patients who are protein-intolerant and develop acute encephalopathy, a short trial of protein restriction may have a role in ameliorating their symptoms without significant loss of total protein turnover. For those with chronic encephalopathy, substitution of nitrogen sources (i.e. increased vegetable or dairy protein, or branched-chain amino acids) should be considered. When considering any such clinical decision, one must take into account other comorbid conditions driving encephalopathy, the patient's hepatic reserve, severity of encephalopathy, and current nutritional status.

References

[1] Seymour CA, Whalen K. Dietary management of hepatic encephalopathy. *BMJ* 1993;318:1364-1365.

[2] Lautz HU, Selberg O, Korber J, Burger M, Muller MF. Protein-calorie malnutrition in liver cirrhosis. *Clin. Investig.* 1992;70:478-486.

[3] SAm. J., Nguyen GC. Protein-calorie malnutrition as a prognostic indicator of mortality among patients hospitalized with cirrhosis and portal hypertension. *Liver Int.* 2009;29:1396-1402.

[4] Mendenhall CL, Tosch T, Weesner RE, Garcia-Pont P, Goldberg SJ, Kiernan T, et al. VA cooperative study on alcoholic hepatitis. II: prognostic significance of protein-calorie malnutrition. *Am. J. Clinc. Nutr.* 1986;43:213-218.
[5] Cabral CM, Burns DL. Low-protein diets for hepatic encephalopathy debunked: let them eat steak. *Nutr. Clin. Practic.* 2011;26:155-159.
[6] Kalman DR, Saltzman JR. Nutrition status predicts survival in cirrhosis. *Nutr. Rev.* 1996;54:217-219.
[7] Merli M, Reggio O, Dally L. Does malnutrition predict survival in cirrhosis? *Hepatology* 1996;23:1041-1046.
[8] O'Brien, R Nutrition in end-stage liver disease: principles and practice. *Gasto* 2008;134:1729-140.
[9] Gundling F, Seidl H, Pehl C, Schmidt T, Schepp W. How close to gastroenterologists follow specific guidelines for nutrition recommendations in liver cirrhosis? A survey of current practice. *Eur. J. Gastroenterol. Hepatol.* 2009;21(7):756-761.
[10] Purnak T, Yilmaz Y. Liver disease and malnurition. *Clin. Gastro* 2013;27(4):619-629.
[11] Petrides AS, Groop LC, Riely CA, DeFronzo RA, et al. Effect of physiologic hyperinsulinemia on glucose and lipid metabolism in cirrhosis. *J. Clin. Invest.* 1991;88:561-570.
[12] Krahenbuhl L, Lang C, Ludes S, Seiler C, Schafer M, Zimmermann A, et al. Reduced hepatic glycogen stores in patients with liver cirrhosis. *Liver Int.* 2003;23:101-109.
[13] Mueller MJ, Bottcher J, Selberg O, Weselmann S, Boker KH, Schwarze M, et al. Hypermetabolism in clinically stable patients with liver cirrhosis. *Am. J. Clin. Nutr.* 1999;69:1066-1068.
[14] Soulsby CT, Morgan MY. Dietary management of hepatic encephalopathy in cirrhotic patients: survey of clinical practice in United Kingdom. *BMJ* 1999;318:1391.
[15] Riordan SM, Williams R. Treatment of hepatic encephalopathy. *N. Eng. J. Med.* 1997;337:413-419.
[16] Phillips GB, Schwartz R, Gabuzda GJ, Davidson CS. The syndrome of impending hepatic coma in patients with cirrhosis of the liver given certain nitrogenous substances. *N. Engl. J. Med.* 1952;247:239-246.
[17] Balo J, Korpassy B. The encephalitis of dogs with Eck fistula fed on meat. *Arch. Pathol.* 1932;13:80-87.
[18] Butterworth RF. The neurobiology of hepatic encephalopathy. *Semin. Liver Dis.* 1996;16:235-244.

[19] Norenberg MD. Astrocytic-ammonia interactions in hepatic encephalopathy. *Semin. Liver Dis.* 1996; 245-253.

[20] Amodio P, Bemeur C, Butterworth R, Cordoba J, Kato A, Montagnese S, et al. The nutritional management of hepatic encephalopathy in patients with cirrhosis: International Society for Hepatic Encephalopathy and Nitrogen Metabolism Consensus. *Hepatology* 2011;58:325-336.

[21] Olde Damink SW. Interorgan ammonia and amino acid metabolism in metabolically stable patients with cirrhosis and a TIPS. *Hepatology* 2002;36:1163-1171.

[22] Merli M, Giusto M, Lucidi C, Giannelli V, Pentassuglio I, Gregorio V, et al. Muscle depletion increases the risk of overt and minimal hepatic encephalopathy: results of a prospective study. *Metab Brain Dis.* 2013;28:281-284.

[23] Cordoba J, Lopez-Hellin J, Planas M, et al. Normal protein diet for episodic hepatic encephalopathy: results of a randomized study. *J. Hepatol.* 2004;41:38-43.

[24] Swart GR, van den Berg JK, van Vuure JK, Rietveld T, Wattimena DL, Frenkel M. Minimum protein requirements in liver cirrhosis determined by nitrogen balance measurements at three levels of protein intake. *Clin. Nutr.* 1989;8(6):329-336.

[25] Gheorghe L, Iacob R, Vandan R, Iacob S, Gheorghe C. Improvement of hepatic encephalopathy using a modified high calorie high protein diet. *Rom. J. Gastroenterol.* 2005;14:231-238.

[26] Blei AT, Cordoba J, Practice Parameters Committee of the American College of Gastroenterology. Hepatic encephalopathy. *Am. J. Gastroenterol.* 2001;58:325-336.

[27] Plauth M, Cabre E, Riggio O, Assis-Camilo M et al. European Society for Parenteral and Enteral Nutrition Guidelines on Enteral Nutrition: Liver disease. *Clin. Nutr.* 2006. 25:285-294.

[28] Bessman AN, Mirick GS. Blood ammonia levels following the ingestion of casein and whole blood. *J. Clin. Invest.* 1958;37:990-998.

[29] Fenton JC, Knight EJ, Humpherson PL. Milk-and-cheese diet in portal-systemic encephalopathy. *Lancet* 1966;1:164-166.

[30] Greenberger NJ, Carley J, Schenker S, et al. Effect of vegetable and animal protein diets in chronic hepatic encephalopathy. *Am. J. Dig. Dis.* 1977;22:845-855.

[31] Weber FL, Mino D, Fresard KM, Banwell JG. Effects of vegetable diets on nitrogen metabolism in cirrhotic subjects. *Gastroenterology* 1985;89:538-544.

[32] Uribe M, Dibildox M, Malpaica S, Guillermo E, VIllallobas A, Nieto L, et al. Beneficial effect of vegetable protein diet supplemented with psyllium plantago in patients with hepatic encephalopathy and diabetes mellitus. *Gastroenterology* 1985;88:901-907.

[33] Vester Boler BM, Faber TA, Bauer LL, Swanson KS, Smiley S, Bechtel PJ et al. Acute satiety response of mammalian, avian and fish proteins in dogs. *Br. J. Nutr.* 2012;107:146-154.

[34] Bosscher D, Breynaert A, Pieters L, Hermans N. Food-based strategies to modulate the composition of the intestinal microbiota and their associated health effects. *J. Physiol. Pharmacol.* 2009;60(Suppl 6):5-11.

[35] Zieve L, Doizaki WM, Zieve J. Synergism between mercaptans and ammonia or fatty acids in the production of coma: a possible role for mercaptans in the pathogenesis of hepatic coma. *J. Lab. Clin. Med.* 1974;83(1):16-28.

[36] de Bruijn KM, Blendis LM, Zilm DH, Carlen PL, Anderson GH, et al. Effects of dietary protein manipulation in subclinical portal systemic encephalopathy. *Gut* 1983;24(1):53-60.

[37] Uribe M, Marquez MA, Garcia Ramos G, Ramos-Uribe MH, Vargas F, Villalobos A. Treatment of chronic portal-systemic encephalopathy with vegetable and animal protein diets. A controlled crossover study. *Dig. Dis. Sci.* 1982;27(12):1109-1116.

[38] Bianchi GP, Marchesni G, Fabbri A, Rondelli A, Bugianesi E, Zoli M, et al. Vegetable verses animal protein diet in cirrhotic patients with chronic encephalopathy. A randomized cross-over comparison. *J. Intern Med.* 1993;233:382-392.

[39] Prakash R, Mullen KD. Mechanisms, diagnosis and management of hepatic encephalopathy. *Nat. Rev. Gastroenterol. Hepatol.* 2010 7:515-525.

[40] James JH, Ziparo V, Jeppsson B, Fischer JE. Hyperammonaemia, plasma amino acid imbalance, and blood-brain amino acid transport: a unified theory of portal-systemic encephalopathy. *Lancet* 1979;2:772-775.

[41] Morgan MY, Milsom JP, Sherlock S. Plasma ratio of valine, leucine and isoleucine to phenylalanine and tyrosine in liver disease. *Gut* 1978;19(11):1068-1073.

[42] Fischer JE, Baldessarini RJ. False neurotransmitters and hepatic failure. *Lancet* 1971;2(7715):75-80.

[43] Marchesini G, Dioguardi FS, Bianchi GP, Zoli M, Bellati G, Roffi L, et al. Long-term oral branched-chain amino acid treatment in chronic

hepatic encephalopathy. A randomized double-blind casein-controlled trial. The Italian Multicenter Study Group. *J. Hepatol.* 1990;11:92-101.

[44] Als-Nielsen B, Koretz RL, Kjaergard LL, Gluud C. Branched-chain amino acids for hepatic encephalopathy. *Cochrane Database Syst. Rev.* 2003;2:CD001939.

[45] Muto Y et al. Effects of oral branched-chain amino acid granules on event-free survival in patients with liver cirrhosis. *Clin. Gastroentrol. Hepatol.* 2005 3:705-713.

[46] Marchesini G, Bianchi G, Merli M, Amodio P, Penella C, Loguercio C et al. Italian BCAA Study Group. Nutritional supplementation with branched-chain amino acids in advanced cirrhosis: a double-blind, randomized trial. *Gastroenterology* 2003;124(7):1792-1801.

[47] Les I, Doval E, Garcia-Martinez R, Planas M, Cardenas G, Gomez P, et al. Effects of branched-chain amino acids supplementation in patients with cirrhosis and a previous episode of hepatic encephalopathy: a randomized study. *Am. J. Gastroentol.* 2011;106:1081-1088.

In: Protein Diets
Editor: Meaghan Hudson

ISBN: 978-1-63463-498-4

Chapter 3

High Protein Weight Loss Diets: Their Impact on Satiety and Intestinal Health

Silvia W. Gratz, Wendy R. Russell and Alexandra M. Johnstone
Rowett Institute of Nutrition and Health, University of Aberdeen, UK

Abstract

Protein is an essential macronutrient in the human diet. In addition to providing essential amino acids to the body, protein has also been linked to inducing the feeling of fullness and satiety. Different sources of protein are traditionally used in the human diet and offer varying amino acid composition. This chapter will summarize work on the implications of the amount and type of protein in the diet to promote the control of hunger and fullness (satiety). Furthermore, evidence regarding the short-term implications of high protein diets on colonic microbiota, fermentation and ultimately intestinal health is presented.

Protein Sources in the Human Diet

The major protein sources in the human diet differ according to geographical region and there is a strong positive relationship between the level of income and the consumption of animal protein. Higher economy countries consume predominantly animal-based protein, where in the rest of the world, plant-based protein is a significant part of the diet. However, in lower economy countries, Latin America and parts of Africa and Asia the demand for meat has increased at a much steeper rate over the last few decades and although overall consumption is still much lower than for industrialized countries, this trend is considered to have an undesirable impact on the environment [1]. Consumption of other animal-derived proteins, milk and dairy products are also increasing at alarming rates worldwide and in this case the rate is much steeper for all non-industrialized countries, with the exception of the transition economies [2].

Of the animal proteins, meat is a high biological value protein (12-35%) with a protein digestibility-corrected amino acid score (PDCAAS) of around 0.9. Meat contains all the essential amino acids and is rich in several micronutrients, particularly iron, selenium, zinc and vitamin B12 [3]. Milk and egg protein have a higher PDCAAS close to 1.0. However, the quality of meat and other animal products can be extremely variable and excessive consumption of animal products is associated with obesity and other co-morbidities, type 2 diabetes mellitus, cardiovascular disease and certain cancers [4].

Plant-based proteins generally have lower digestibility compared to animal proteins (PDCAAS < 0.75). Individually plants are generally not a complete source of amino acids, lacking in particular lysine (cereals), cysteine and methionine (legumes). To achieve an essential level of amino acids these foods require to be consumed in combination. Despite this, plant-based protein sources are required to meet increasing worldwide demand for proteins, and could contribute towards improving human health and alleviating the threat imposed to the environment by current agricultural practice in higher-economy countries i.e. dependence on fossil energy and harmful emissions [5]. Of the land-plants, legumes have the highest protein content (up to 40%), with soya bean currently being the most important commercial source [6]. Other key sources are pea, chickpea and lupin. Pea contains 20-30% protein, is easily dehulled and often used in the form of protein fractions and isolates [7]. Chickpea is a particularly important crop in the Indian sub-continent and contains around 20-25% protein. Lupin has exceptionally high protein content (35-40%) and white lupin is consumed directly as a food throughout Europe and in Australia [8]. Although lower in protein content (up to 17%), the cereals, especially wheat and rice are the most important food crops worldwide. Wheat contains approx. 8-15% protein and provides the largest contribution of protein to the human diet world-wide. Rice has the lowest protein content (< 10%), but is the second most important cereal crop, mostly being grown and consumed in Asia. Sorghum, maize and barley are also important protein-rich cereals containing around 9-17%, 9-12% and 8-15% respectively [9]. Other sources of plant-based protein in the diet include nuts and tubers. Tubers such as potato are generally low in protein (approx. 1%), but protein isolates from potato can be a nutritionally valuable source [10].

EFFECT OF DIETARY PROTEIN ON SATIETY AND WEIGHT LOSS

The protein composition of an individual's diet can be considered in different ways, as the absolute amount of the protein (grams), the % of total energy (calories) as protein or the amount of protein ingested per kg of body weight. Normal protein intake in the UK is approximately 16% of energy intake [11] for a sedentary adult, which is approximately 64-88g/d at energy balance for females and males, respectively. The guidelines from the US Institute of Medicine allow for the inclusion of higher amounts of protein than previously recommended in a healthy diet [12]. Thus, the acceptable protein distribution was set to 5-20% of calories for children aged 1-3 yr, 10-30% for children aged 3-18 yr and 10-35% for adults. There is no general consensus as to what a 'high' protein diet is and the food industry use the term 'protein-enriched' for 20% protein from calories [13]. In the developed world, we currently eat in excess of our calorie and protein requirements contributing to the overweight and obesity problem. Over eating energy will often mean over consuming protein as an absolute amount (g). This will not improve satiety feedback to curb consumption. In the context of high-protein diets for weight loss, this can be considered a diet that contains a greater proportion of protein (%) from energy. Increasing protein % will invoke an appetite response to decrease *ad libitum* energy intake.

High protein diets reported in weight loss studies often include around 30% of energy intake as protein. There are many variants such as the Zone diet [14] and the CSIRO diet [15]. In general, protein as a percentage of energy is doubled from 15% to 30%. Note, this does not mean that absolute protein intake (g) is doubled, as energy intake is reduced, with only a 20% increase in the actual amount (g) of protein. It is not clear how much protein is required to induce or maximize protein-induced satiety or whether there is a relationship with the energy density of the diet. Future research could focus on these areas. Both the safety and efficacy [16] of high-protein weight loss diets have been questioned, particularly in combination with low-carbohydrate advice [17]. This has been recently reviewed [18] with growing evidence to support the use of high-protein, moderate-carbohydrate diets as a dietary tool to achieve weight loss (e.g. 30% protein, 30% fat and 40% carbohydrate).

Short-term Effects of Protein on Appetite

Protein is more satiating than carbohydrate and fat in the short term (within day), over 24 h and in the medium term (several days or weeks) [19]. In general, studies that examine subjective hunger and fullness after a pre-load test meal or drink may also include a period of monitoring food and energy intake at the next eating episode, conducted within one day. In general, in the short term feeding period, 'fast' proteins are more satiating than 'slow' proteins, and animal protein induces a higher thermogenesis than vegetable protein, (where ‘fast’ and ‘slow’ refers to the speed of digestion and absorption of the protein source) [19]. Halton & Hu [20] have summarized the main findings, that of the 14 studies that compared high protein to at least one other macronutrient, 11 found that the protein preload significantly increased subjective ratings of satiety. Other studies that have used nose-clips and liquid format [21, 22] have not found effects of high-protein meals suggesting a role in sensory characteristics in promoting satiety. Veldhorstet et al. have published many preloading studies that suggest that high-protein diets are more satiating in comparison to normal protein meals, when fed at iso-energetic amounts [23-25]. In summary, the evidence supports the conclusion that meals higher in protein tend to increase satiety when compared to meals lower in protein, at least in the short term.

In the medium term, in studies conducted over a few days, the higher post-absorptive satiety and thermogenesis are sustained irrespective of the protein source [20]. There is no clear consensus that one type of protein is more satiating than another. Overall, the weight of evidence suggests that higher protein intakes cause a decreased subsequent energy intake, although the results are not entirely consistent. It appears that, the closer the methodology is to real life situations (real food vs. liquid, sense of taste unaltered, free living vs. whole body calorimeter), the more likely it is for protein to exert a significant decrease in subsequent energy intake [20]. There are, however, some methodological issues concerning this type of research. Satiety appears to be influenced by a wide variety of factors including palatability, food mass, energy density, fiber content/type and glycemic index. When using real foods, it is difficult, if not impossible to control for all of these influences at the same time while still delivering different amounts of protein [20].

Longer Term Effects of Protein on Satiety

Most of the studies on protein are conducted with an end point to assess appetite and food intake and a view to influencing body weight. High-protein diets provide a potential benefit of improved compliance during weight loss attempts. Skov et al. [26] have shown larger weight-loss benefits at six months on a high-protein weight-loss regime. Furthermore, groups consuming a high-protein, moderate-carbohydrate diet have an increased likelihood of maintaining weight loss at 12 months and beyond, with improvements in cardiovascular risk factors and minimal risk of side effects [27, 28]. In a 12 month study, Due et al. [29] reported substantially greater compliance in subjects consuming a higher-protein diet (25% protein of energy) with an 8% drop out rate compared with subjects on a low protein diet (12% energy) with a 28% drop out. Indeed, the recent extensive EU-wide Diogenes trial [30] examined low and high protein diets with low and high glycemic index (GI) components. Specifically, of the five popular diet types tested, a high-protein, low-GI diet provided the greatest opportunity for weight loss maintenance. The dropout rate was lower in the groups that were assigned to high-protein diets and the groups that were assigned to low-GI diets than in the group that was assigned to the diet that was low in protein and had a high-GI (26.4% and 25.6%, respectively, vs. 37.4%; P = 0.02 and P = 0.01 for the high-protein groups, low-GI groups and low-protein, low-GI groups, respectively).

In weight loss studies, free-living subjects feeding *ad libitum* from high-protein diets show a weight loss of around ~1kg a week [31, 32] which is consistent with current dietary advice on rate of weight loss from health professionals [33]. As a result of the weight loss, there are significant improvements in body composition, blood pressure, and bio-markers of health. The reduction in body fat mass (kg) and maintenance of lean mass (kg) during weight loss has been reported previously by other authors and, in part, is related to the protein enriched composition of the diet [34]. In a recent meta regression, Krieger et al. [35] examined 87 short term studies and found that protein intakes of >1.05 g/kg of actual (rather than desirable) body weight were associated with 0.6 kg better retention of lean mass, and in studies greater than 12 weeks in duration, this increased to 1.2 kg. In studies that used a carbohydrate intake of less than 35-41% there was a 2 kg greater loss of fat mass, and this was accompanied by a 0.7 kg greater loss of lean mass. In studies of 12 weeks or more this increased to 5.6 kg and 1.7 kg, respectively. Several studies have also looked at body composition to test the hypothesis that higher protein diets spare the lean body mass of those on energy restricted diets. Most found greater fat loss with the high protein diets in comparison to the lower protein diets, but fewer reported this to be statistically significant, probably a function of body composition techniques and small study sizes [35]. In general, it is accepted that a reduced-carbohydrate, high protein diet is associated with better fat loss and relatively less lean mass loss.

Follow up of Weight Regain after High Protein Weight Loss Diet

Several groups have examined regain of weight following a high protein diet with similar outcomes. Lejeune et al. [36] report a 20% increase in protein intake (through an unmatched supplement) during weight maintenance, after a four-week weight-loss period and reduced weight regain by 50% over the subsequent three months. After six months on a weight-maintenance diet, there was a weight regain of 0.8 kg (high protein group) vs. 3.0 kg (control group) ($p < 0.05$) and during follow-up of one year after the weight loss program, these figures were 1.0 kg vs. 3.9 kg ($p < 0.05$). Claessens et al. [37] report a similar effect using a matched casein supplement over 12 weeks of weight maintenance, which amounted to a differential of 2.2 kg of fat. Layman et al. [38] found that a weight loss diet that had double the amount of protein (1.6 g/kg vs 0.8 g/kg) led to better body composition at both four months and 12 months, especially in those participants who lost more than 10% of their body weight over this period. It is the aforementioned large-scale 'Diogenes' trial that provides the most convincing data on the benefits of high-protein, low-GI diets for longer-term weight control [30]. Specifically, weight regain was 0.93 kg less for the 773 participants on a high-protein diet than for those on a low-protein diet and 0.95 kg less in the groups on a low-GI diet compared to those on a high-GI diet [30]. These data support the use of high-protein, moderate-carbohydrate diets to achieve weight control. Thus, evidence indicates that a relatively high-protein intake sustains weight maintenance by (i) favouring regain of fat free mass at the cost of fat mass at a similar physical activity level, (ii) reducing the energy efficiency with respect to the body mass regained, and (iii) increasing satiety.

Taken together, relative high-protein diets, offered *ad libitum*, whereby the absolute amount of protein as consumed before dieting is sustained, promote weight loss as well as weight maintenance. It remains to be assessed whether and how types of protein contribute differently to this phenomenon.

Type of Protein and Amount of Protein

Specific types of protein may affect satiety by different mechanisms. To date there has been no clear-cut assessment of protein sources that include fed to energy balance or weight loss conditions in lean or overweight men and women and this may be due to methodological and/or practical problems conducting these studies. Some studies, but not all, demonstrate a higher satiating effect of whey and fish proteins compared with other protein sources. The evidence from intervention studies comparing the effects of different protein sources on body weight is inconclusive. A dose dependent satiating effect of protein has been shown, with a range of concentrations of protein offered acutely in a single meal, to subjects who are in energy balance and weight stable (e.g. 39-41). In addition, persistent protein-induced satiety has been shown when a high-protein diet was given for 24 h up to several days (e.g. 42-44). Hall et al. [45] report a significantly lower energy intake following a whey protein preload compared with casein preload. However, when a buffet meal was offered at 90 min after the preloads, it was possibly too soon for casein to be a realistic and sensitive time-point. Bowen et al. [46, 47] compared energy intake, ghrelin, and cholecystokinin after different carbohydrate and protein preloads in overweight men. No effect from different proteins i.e. casein and whey was observed, yet the high-protein meals induced a larger satiating effect compared with the high-carbohydrate beverages. Furthermore, it was noted that different appetite regulatory hormone responses to various dietary proteins, i.e. after whey, soy, or gluten preload, by differences in body mass index status despite similar reductions in *ad libitum* energy intake [48]. Lang et al. [49] did not observe significant differences in energy intake or macronutrient intake at dinner (7 hr after lunch) or over 24 h following a test lunch with casein, gelatin, or soy protein. Neither did they observe significantly different effects of egg albumin, casein, gelatin, soy, pea, or wheat gluten on appetite scores or energy intake [50]. Veldhorst et al. [23-25] conducted a series of studies on effects of different types of protein (casein, soy, whey, and whey without GMP: Glycomacropeptide) ingestion, each in two different quantities (10% and 25% of energy from the single protein type). It was discovered that outcomes differed due to the type or quantity of protein intake, or both. For instance, with whey as a single protein in a subject specifically standardized custard breakfast, energy intake at lunch, 3 h after a breakfast with whey still containing GMP compared to energy intake after a breakfast with whey without GMP, was decreased by 13% irrespective of the whey protein content being 10 or 25% of energy in the custard breakfast. Therefore, there are limited data to support clear differences in satiating properties between different protein types are shown, mainly due to the design of the study, using not just one single protein, or to the timing of feeding [51].

Although it is generally noted that timing is an important consideration concerning protein kinetics and appetite [52], there is limited data to support that amino acid metabolism is the strongest cue for appetite by the groups that have attempted to link plasma amino acid profiles with hunger ratings. Westerterp-Plantenga [24] investigated the dynamic relationship between appetite, type of protein, plasma amino acid profile and gut hormones, for soy protein, without much enlightenment. Metabolites, including certain amino acids, contribute to the perception of postprandial satiety [19]. Mellinkoff suggested in 1956 a relationship between serum amino acid concentration and fluctuations in appetite [53]. Since amino acid concentrations were correlated with a reduction in appetite, Mellinkoff believed these to be connected to a 'satiety center' in the brain. In this hypothesis, the center is sensitive to serum amino acid levels and once levels reach a certain point, hunger would cease. It would seem to make sense that the control of amino acids would be a priority considering their importance for tissue growth and maintenance, coupled with their potential for toxicity at very high levels. With respect to central regulation, Faipoux et al. [54] have discussed that that protein-induced satiety was related to vagal feedback to (i) the nucleus tractus solitarius in the brainstem, where it represents satiety at almost a reflex level, and (ii) the hypothalamus, where it suppresses feelings of hunger. It may be the subjective psychological hunger rating system is not sufficiently sensitive to pick up such acute changes in physiology (see more discussion below).

It is worth mentioning the review of Gilbert et al. [55] considering the effect of protein source on body composition during weight loss, aside from the appetite effects. High-protein diets have beneficial effects on body fat regulation, but the difference in effect of various types of protein is not known. Animal proteins, especially those from dairy, seem to support better muscle protein synthesis during weight reduction regimes in comparison to plant proteins because they contain all essential amino acids and are generally well digested. This could potentially enhance energy expenditure, but no conclusion can be drawn from the scant evidence [55]. However, body composition was not evaluated precisely in these studies and the literature is still incomplete (e.g. comparative data are missing for legumes and nuts). Protein intake enhances energy expenditure, satiety and fat loss, but there is no clear evidence to indicate whether there is a difference in the effect size dependent on the source of the protein, i.e. from animal- or plant-based foods.

Further research is warranted to investigate the mechanistic basis for protein induced satiety (PIS), particularly in studies where negative energy balance (dieting or weight loss) is induced, when PIS effects are likely to be amplified. The amount of protein (grams or proportion), type, timing and interactions with other interventions (e.g. exercise or energy density) are still to be optimized. Protein remains a promising dietary tool to control appetite during weight loss.

EFFECT OF DIETARY PROTEIN ON INTESTINAL HEALTH

Colonic Protein Breakdown

Protein digestion and absorption in the human small intestine is very efficient with about 90% of dietary protein being absorbed and only 10% reaching the colon. The exact amount is mainly determined by the amount and type of dietary protein consumed. Approximately 12-18 g/day of protein reaches the human colon and comprises a mixture of residual dietary protein and enzymes secreted in the upper part of the intestine [55]. Colonic microbiota primarily utilize carbohydrates as substrates for fermentation and growth and protein is less efficiently used as an energy substrate [56]. Proteolytic activity as well as fermentation of amino acids as an energy source occurs predominantly in the distal part of the human colon where carbohydrates are scarce and the luminal pH is near neutral [57]. Important proteolytic bacteria in human fecal samples include *Bacteroides* as well as *Propionibacteria, Streptococcus, Clostridia (e.g. C. perfringens), Bacillus, and Staphylococcus* species [58]. Many bacterial species preferably ferment amino acids including: *Peptococci*, *Acidaminococcus*, *Veillonella*, and some *Fusobacteria*, *Eubacteria* and *Clostridia* species [59]. Furthermore, many saccharolytic bacteria use amino acids and peptides as nitrogen sources [60].

Protein Fermentation Products

The metabolic profile of amino acid fermentation is more diverse compared to carbohydrate fermentation, including organic acids, ammonia, amines, phenols, indoles and the gases H_2 and CO_2 [61, 62]. Many of these metabolites are linked to negative health effects for the gut epithelium and the host. Deamination is the most important route of amino acid fermentation in the human colon utilizing approximately 30% of substrates. This results in the production of ammonia and organic acids including the major short chain fatty acids (SCFA) acetate, propionate, butyrate and the branched chain fatty acids (BCFA) iso-butyrate and iso-valerate [60]. These BCFA derive from branched-chain amino acids valine, isoleucine and leucine [59, 63] and are good fecal indicators for protein fermentation. Fecal ammonia concentration varies from 12-30 mM in humans [64]. Ammonia is rapidly absorbed from the gut via the portal vein, metabolized in the liver and excreted in urine as urea. In the gut, ammonia alters morphology and metabolism of intestinal cells and may act as tumor promoter. Deamination of aromatic amino acids releases phenols and indoles (p-cresol and phenylproprionate from tyrosine; phenylacetate from phenylalanine; indole propionate and indole acetate from tryptophan). Phenolic compounds are rapidly absorbed and excreted mainly as urinary p-cresol (> 90%). Bacterial decarboxylation of amino acid is another route of fermentation resulting in numerous amines including agamatine, tyramine, pyrrolidine, histamine, piperidine, cadaverine, prutrescine and 5-hydroxytryptamine [65]. Amines are detoxified efficiently by mono- and diamine oxidases in the gut tissue and liver and their direct toxicity is not well understood. However, they can act as precursors in the formation of nitrosamines such as N-nitrosodimethylamine, a probable human carcinogen. Sulphate reducing bacteria in the human gut produce hydrogen sulfide (H_2S), a noxious chemical derived from dietary inorganic sulphur and sulphur-containing amino acids (methionine, cysteine, cystine and taurine) [66]. Colonic sulphide is suggested to be linked to the development of inflammatory bowel disease and ulcerative colitis [59].

Diet Composition Influences Protein Fermentation

Studies directly assessing the effect of dietary protein on colonic microbiota composition are rare and most studies assess fermentation products. In human flora associated rats, feeding diets enriched with pea protein or soy protein isolates showed similar patterns of fermentation metabolites in caecal contents, whereas rats on a meat diet showed lower total SCFA and butyrate levels, higher BCFA, ammonia levels and higher pH compared to pea protein fed animals [67]. Increased intake of milk protein increased BCFA (twofold) and ammonia (5.5 fold) in colonic contents of rats compared to low milk protein diet [68].

Dietary protein and especially red meat have long been studied in terms of their contribution to increased risk of colorectal cancer in humans. The world cancer research fund (WCRF) has concluded that the scientific evidence suggests a convincing link between increased red and processed meat consumption and increased risk of colorectal cancer [69]. The suggested mechanism involved includes the endogenous production of N-nitroso compounds (including carcinogenic nitrosamines) as a result of colonic bacterial activity. Red meat has been clearly shown to increase endogenous formation of nitrosamines, and WCRF recommends limited intake of red meat to no more than 500g/week (cooked weight) in order to limit the risk of colorectal cancer. Furthermore, high meat diets (600g/d) have been shown to increase faecal sulphide concentration in humans [66].

Carbohydrate supply and fermentation have been suggested to limit proteolytic production of toxic metabolites through enhancing bacterial proteosynthesis [57]. Arabinoxylan-oligosaccharide supplementation has been shown *in vitro* to decrease production of phenol and p-cresol [70] and authors suggest a shift in fermentation activity rather than microbial community. In mice, the inclusion of resistant starch into a high red meat diet was shown to increase SCFAs and decrease proteolytic metabolites (Ammonia, phenol, p-cresol) [71]. Similarly, resistant starch counteracted the increased fermentation of indigestible potato protein (measured as fecal BCFA and urinary phenol and p-cresol) in rats [72]. In humans, shifting from a low meat to a high meat diet increases fecal pH, fecal ammonia and fecal N-nitroso compounds, but incorporation of RS into high meat diets only lowered fecal pH; ammonia and N-nitroso compounds remained high and SCFA were not measured [73]. A randomized placebo controlled human intervention trial showed that supplementing healthy volunteers with prebiotics (oligofructose enriched inulin) decreased proteolytic metabolites in urine (15N and p-cresols) and also increased fecal bacterial N15 content, suggesting increased bacterial proliferation as a result of increased carbohydrate availability in the colon [74].

Although high-protein diets offer an effective method of weight loss in obese individuals, there is a concern that inadequate fiber in the diet could impact on the normal function of the human gut. In a carefully controlled human study, high-protein (138 g/d)-low-carbohydrate diets (8.8 or 14 g/d) were compared with a weight maintenance diet containing adequate protein and fiber. After four weeks, consumption of the high-protein low-carbohydrate diets resulted in a significant decrease in cancer-protective compounds (short chain fatty acids and anti-inflammatory phenolic compounds) and increased concentrations of hazardous N-nitroso compounds in the gut. Long-term adherence to such diets is likely to increase risk of colonic disease [75]. Further dietary intervention studies in obese volunteers have shown that fecal N-nitroso compounds are driven by red meat intake, but a lack of dietary fiber intake further enhances N-nitroso compound production in humans [76]. Similarly, colonic amino acid fermentation (measured as fecal BCFA) is negatively correlated with dietary carbohydrate intake, but unrelated to dietary protein [77]. In summary, these findings suggest that shifts in colonic fermentation towards amino acid breakdown in humans are driven by both high dietary protein (and meat) intakes and a lack of dietary carbohydrate.

Conclusion

In conclusion, protein remains a promising dietary tool to control appetite during weight loss.

Further research is warranted to investigate the mechanistic basis for protein induced satiety (PIS), as well as the amount of protein and the type, timing and interactions with other interventions (e.g. exercise or energy density) are still to be optimized. In terms of intestinal health, a clear preference has to be given to balancing protein enriched diets with moderate amounts of non-digestible carbohydrates in order to prevent shifts in intestinal microbiota and fermentation products towards a detrimental effect. From an environmental point of view, ever increasing meat and dairy consumption has environmental implications, such as greenhouse gas emissions, climate change and land use. Hence more diverse and sustainable sources of protein have to be explored to meet the global demand.

Acknowledgment

The Rowett Institute of Nutrition and Health receives funding from the Scottish Government, Rural and Environment Science and Analytical Services Division (RESAS).

References

[1] Fukagawa N. K. & Yu Y.-M. (2009) *Nutrition and Metabolism of Proteins and Amino Acids.* In: Gibney M. J., Lanham-New S. A., Dassidy A., Vorseer H. H. (Eds), Introduction to Human Nutrition (2nd Edition), p 49-73. Chichester, UK. Wiley-Blackwell.

[2] Bruinsma J. ed. *World agriculture: Towards 2015/2030.* An FAO perspective. Rome, Food and Agriculture Organization of the United Nations/London, Earthscan, 2003.

[3] Pereira P. M. C. C. & Vicente A. F. R. B. (2013) Meat nutritional composition and nutritive role in the human diet. *Meat Sci* 93, 586-592.

[4] Chan D. S. M. et al. (2011) Red and Processed Meat and Colorectal Cancer Incidence: Meta-Analysis of Prospective Studies. *Plos One,* 6, 20456.

[5] Aiking H. et al. (2011) Future Protein Supply. *Trends Food Sci Technol,* 22, 112-120.

[6] Johnson L. A. et al. (2008) *Soybeans.* Chemistry, production, processing, and utilization. USA: AOCS press.

[7] Boyle J. I. et al. (2010) Comparison of the functional properties of pea, chickpea and lentil protein concentrates processed using ultrafiltration and isoelectric precipitation techniques. *Food Res Internat,* 43, 537-546.

[8] Evans A. J. et al. (1993) Carbohydrate-composition of cotyledons and hulls of cultivars of Lupinusangustifolius from Western-Australia. *J Sci Food Agric,* 61, 189-194.

[9] Day L. (2013) Proteins from land plants Potential resources for human nutrition and food security. *Trends Food Sci Technol,* 32, 25-42.

[10] Bartova V. & Barta J. (2009) Chemical composition and nutritional value of protein concentrates isolated from potato (Solanum tuberosum L.) fruit juice by precipitation with ethanol or ferric chloride. *J Agric Food Chem,* 57, 9028-9034.

[11] Henderson L. et al. (2003) *The National Diet & Nutrition Survey: Adults aged 19 to 64 years.* Volumes 1-4: Stationery Office, Norwich: HMSO.

[12] Trumbo P. et al. (2002) Dietary reference intakes for energy, carbohydrate, fiber, fat, fatty acids, cholesterol, protein and amino acids. Food and Nutrition Board, Institute of Medicine, The National Academies, USA. *J Am Diet Assoc,* 102, 1621-1630.

[13] Westerterp-Plantenga M. S. (2007) How are normal, high- or low-protein diets defined? *Ann Nutr Metab,* 51(Supp l1), 6.

[14] Gardner C. D. et al. (2007) Comparison of the Atkins, Zone, Ornish, and LEARN diets for change in weight and related risk factors among overweight premenopausal women: The A to Z Weight Loss Study: A randomized trial. *JAMA,* 297, 969-977.

[15] Wyld B. et al. (2010) The CSIRO Total Wellbeing Diet Book 1: Sociodemographic differences and impact on weight loss and well-being in Australia. *Public Health Nutr,* 13, 2105-2110.

[16] St Jeor S. T. et al. (2001) Dietary protein and weight reduction: A statement for healthcare professionals from the Nutrition Committee of the Council on Nutrition, Physical Activity, and Metabolism of the American Heart Association. *Circulation,* 104, 1869-1874.

[17] Astrup A. (2005) Satiating power of protein: A key to obesity prevention? *Am J ClinNutr,* 82, 1-2.

[18] Johnstone, (2012) Safety and efficacy of high protein diets for weight loss. *Proc Nutr Soc,* 71, 339-349.

[19] Veldhorst M. et al. (2008) Protein-induced satiety: Effects and mechanisms of different proteins. *Physio lBehaviour,* 94(2), 300-307.

[20] Halton T. L. & Hu F. B. (2004) The effects of high protein diets on thermogenesis, satiety and weight loss: A critical review. *J Am Coll Nutr,* 23(5), 373-385.

[21] Geliebter A. A. (1979) Effects of equicaloric loads of protein, fat, and carbohydrate on food intake in the rat and man. *Physiol Behaviour,* 22(2), 267-273.

[22] De Graaf C. et al. (1992) Short term effects of different amounts of protein, fats and carbohydrate on satiety. *Am J ClinNutr,* 55, 33-38.

[23] Veldhorst M. A. et al. (2009) Dose-dependent satiating effect of whey relative to casein or soy. *Physiol Behav,* 96, 675-682.

[24] Veldhorst M. A. et al. (2009) Effects of high and normal soy protein breakfasts on satiety and subsequent energy intake, including amino acid and 'satiety' hormone responses. *Eur J Nutr,* 48, 92-100.

[25] Veldhorst M. A. et al. (2009) Effects of complete whey-protein breakfasts versus whey without GMP-breakfasts on energy intake and satiety. *Appetite,* 52, 388-395.

[26] Skov A. R. et al. (1999) Randomized trial on protein vs. carbohydrate in ad libitum fat reduced diet for the treatment of obesity. *Int J Obes* (Lond), 23, 1170-1177.

[27] Clifton P. M. (2006) Science behind weight loss diets: A brief review. *Aust Fam Physician,* 35, 580-582.

[28] Clifton P. M. (2006) Value of high-protein diet is clearer than drawbacks. *Nature,* 439, 266.

[29] Due A. et al. (2004) Effect of normal-fat diets, either medium or high in protein, on body weight in overweight subjects: A randomized 1-year trial. *Int J Obes Relat Metab Disord* 28, 1283-1290.

[30] Larsen T. M. et al. (2010) The Diet, Obesity and Genes (Diogenes) Dietary Study in eight European countries: A comprehensive design for long-term intervention. *Obes Rev* 11, 76-91.

[31] Johnstone A. M. et al. (2008) Hunger and appetite response to a high-protein ketogenic diet in obese men feeding ad libitum. *Am J Clin Nutr* 87, 44-55.

[32] Johnstone A. M. et al. (2011) Effects of a high-protein, low-carbohydrate weight loss diet on antioxidant status, endothelial function and plasma indices of cardio-metabolic profile. *Br J Nutr* 106, 282-291.

[33] British Dietetic Association, www.bda.uk.com.

[34] Wycherley T. P. et al. (2010) A high-protein diet with resistance exercise training improves weight loss and body composition in overweight and obese patients with type 2 diabetes. *Diabetes Care* 33, 969-976.

[35] Krieger J. W. et al. (2006) Effects of variation in protein and carbohydrate intake on body mass and composition during energy restriction: A meta-regression. *Am J Clin Nutr,* 83, 260-274.

[36] Lejeune M. P. et al. (2005) Additional protein intake limits weight regain after weight loss in humans. *Br J Nutr,* 93, 281-289.

[37] Claessens M. et al. (2009) Effect of a low-fat, high-protein or high-carbohydrate ad libitum diet on weight loss maintenance and metabolic risk factors. *Int J Obes* (Lond), 33, 296-304.

[38] Layman D. K. et al. (2009) Moderate-protein diet produces sustained weight loss and long-term changes in body composition and blood lipids in obese adults. *J Nutr* 139(3), 514-521.

[39] Williams et al. (2006) High protein high fibre snack bars reduce food intake and improve short term glucose and insulin profiles compared with high fat snack bars. *Asia Pac J Clin Nutr,* 15(4), 443-50.

[40] Boelsma E. et al. (2010) Measures of postprandial wellness after single intake of two protein-carbohydrate meals. *Appetite,* 54(3), 456-464.

[41] Lorenzen J. et al. (2012) Effect of milk proteins on appetite regulation and diet-induced thermogenesis. *Eur J ClinNutr,* 66(5), 622-627.

[42] Due A. et al. (2004) Effect of normal-fat diets, either medium or high in protein, on body weight in overweight subjects: A randomized 1-year trial. *Int J Obes Relat Metab Disord* 28(10), 1283-1290.

[43] Noakes M. et al. (2005) Effect of an energy-restricted, high-protein, low-fat diet relative to a conventional high-carbohydrate, low-fat diet on weight loss, body composition, nutritional status, and markers of cardiovascular health in obese women. *Am J Clin Nutr,* 81(6), 1298-1306.

[44] Jakubowicz D. et al. (2012) Meal timing and composition influence ghrelin levels, appetite scores and weight loss maintenance in overweight and obese adults. *Steroids,* 77(SI4), 323-331.

[45] Hall et al. (2003) Casein and whey exert different effects on plasma amino acid profiles, gastrointestinal hormone secretion and appetite. *Br J Nutr,* 89(2), 239-248.

[46] Bowen J. et al. (2006a) Energy intake, ghrelin, and cholecystokinin after different carbohydrate and protein preloads in overweight men. *J Clin Endocrin Metab,* 91(4), 1477-1483.

[47] Bowen J. et al. (2007) Appetite hormones and energy intake in obese men after consumption of fructose, glucose and whey protein beverages. *Int J Obesity,* 31(11), 1696-1703.

[48] Bowen J. et al. (2006b) Appetite regulatory hormone responses to various dietary proteins differ by body mass index status despite similar reductions in ad libitum energy intake. *J Clin Endocrin Metab,* 91(8), 2914-2919.

[49] Lang V. et al. (1999) Varying the protein source in mixed meal modifies glucose, insulin and glucagon kinetics in healthy men, has weak effects on subjective satiety and fails to affect food intake. *Eur J Clin Nutr,* 53(12), 959-965.

[50] Lang V. et al. (1998) Satiating effect of proteins in healthy subjects: Comparison of egg albumin, casein, gelatin, soy protein, pea protein, and wheat gluten. *Am J Clin Nutr,* 67(6), 1197-1204.

[51] Chungchunlam S. M. S. et al. (2012) Effect of time of consumption of preloads on measures of satiety in healthy normal weight women. *Appetite,* 59(2), 281-288.

[52] Luhovyy B. L. et al. (2007) Whey proteins in the regulation of food intake and satiety. *J Am Coll Nutr,* 26(6), 704S-712S.

[53] Mellinkoff S. M. et al. (1997) Relationship between serum amino acid concentration and fluctuations in appetite. *Obesity Res,* 5(4), 381-384.

[54] Faipoux R. et al. (2008) Proteins activate satiety-related neuronal pathways in the brainstem and hypothalamus of rats. *J Nutr,* 138(6), 1172-1178.

[55] Gilbert J. A. et al. (2011) Effect of proteins from different sources on body composition. *Nutr Metab Cardiovasc Dis,* 21, Suppl. 2, B16-23.

[56] Cummings J. H. & Macfarlane G. T. (1997) Role of intestinal bacteria in nutrient metabolism. *J Parenter Enteral Nutr,* 21(6), 357-365.

[57] Caballero-Franco C. et al. (2007) The VSL#3 probiotic formula induces mucin gene expression and secretion in colonic epithelial cells. *Am J Physiol Gastrointest Liver Physiol,* 292(1), G315-322.

[58] Bernalier-Donadille A. (2010) Fermentative metabolism by the human gut microbiota. *Gastroenterologie Clinique et Biologique,* 34, S16-S22.

[59] Macfarlane S. & Macfarlane G. T. (1995) *Proteolysis and Amino Acid Fermentation.* In: Gibson G. R. & Macfarlane G. T. (Eds), Human Colonic Bacteria: Role in Nutrition, Physiology and Pathology, p. 75-100, CRC Press Inc.

[60] Macfarlane G. T. & Macfarlane S. (1997) Human colonic microbiota: Ecology, physiology and metabolic potential of intestinal bacteria. *Scand J Gastroenterol Suppl,* 222, 3-9.

[61] Cummings J. H. & Macfarlane G. T. (1991) Control and consequences of bacterial fermentation in the human colon. *J Appl Bacteriol,* 70(6), 443-459.

[62] Scott K. P. et al. (2013) Influence of diet on the gut microbiota. *Pharmacol Res* 69(1), 52-60.

[63] Hamer H. M. et al. (2011) Functional analysis of colonic bacterial metabolism: Relevant to health? *Am J Physiol Gastrointest Liver Physiol,* 302(1), G1-9.

[64] Rasmussen H. S. et al. (1988) Degradation of amino acids to short-chain fatty acids in humans. An *in vitro* study. *Scand J Gastroenterol,* 23(2), 178-182.

[65] Smith E. A. & Macfarlane G. T. (1996) Studies on Amino Production in the Human Colon: Enumeration of Amine forming Bacteria and Physiological Effects of Carbohydrate and pH. *Anaerobe,* 2, 285-297.

[66] Magee E. A. et al. (2000) Contribution of dietary protein to sulfide production in the large intestine: *In vitro* and a controlled feeding study in humans. *Am J Clin Nutr,* 72(6), 1488-1494.

[67] Lhoste E. F. et al. (1998) Physiological effects of a pea protein isolate in gnotobiotic rats: Comparison with a soybean isolate and meat. *Ann Nutr Metab,* 42(1), 44-54.

[68] Andriamihaja M. et al. (2010) Colon luminal content and epithelial cell morphology markedly modified in rats fed with a high-protein diet. *Am J Physiol Gastrointest Liver Physiol,* 299(5), G1030-1037.

[69] World Cancer Research Fund (2011) *Food, nutrition, physical activity and the prevention of cancer: A global perspective* (Continuous Update Project), AICR Washington DC.

[70] Sanchez J. I. et al. (2009) Arabinoxylan-oligosaccharides (AXOS) affect the protein/carbohydrate fermentation balance and microbial population dynamics of the Simulator of Human Intestinal Microbial Ecosystem. *Microb Biotechnol,* 2(1), 101-13.

[71] Winter J. et al. (2011) Inhibition by resistant starch of red meat-induced promutagenic adducts in mouse colon. *Cancer Prev Res* (Phila), 4(11), 1920-1928.

[72] Le Leu R. K. et al. (2007) Effect of dietary resistant starch and protein on colonic fermentation and intestinal tumourigenesis in rats. *Carcinogenesis* 28(2), 240-245.

[73] Silvester K. R. et al. (1997) Effect of meat and resistant starch on fecal excretion of apparent N-nitroso compounds and ammonia from the human large bowel. *Nutr Cancer* 29(1), 13-23.

[74] De Preter V. et al. (2007) Effects of Lactobacillus casein Shirota, Bifidobacterium breve, and oligofructose-enriched inulin on colonic nitrogen-protein metabolism in healthy humans. *Am J Physiol Gastrointest Liver Physiol* 292(1), G358-368.

[75] Russell W. R. et al. (2011) High-protein, reduced-carbohydrate weight-loss diets promote metabolite profiles likely to be detrimental to colonic health. *Am J Clin Nutr,* 93(5), 1062-1072.

[76] Holtrop G. et al. (2012) Diet composition is associated with endogenous formation of N-nitroso compounds in obese men. *J Nutr* 142(9), 1652-1658.

[77] Gratz S. W. et al. (2014) Influence of dietary carbohydrate and protein on colonic fermentation and endogenous formation of N-nitroso compounds. *Proc Nutr Soc* 73 (OCE3).

In: Protein Diets
Editor: Meaghan Hudson

ISBN: 978-1-63463-498-4

Chapter 4

DIETARY PROTEIN: SOURCES, METABOLISM AND RECOMMENDATION FOR POULTRY AND SWINE

Verônica Maria Pereira Bernardino*[*1], Carolina Fontes Prezotto[2], Cinthia Maria Carlos Pereira[3] and Camila Meneghetti[3]

[1]PhD in Non-ruminant Nutrition by the Federal University of Lavras – UFLA, Lavras, Minas Gerais, Brazil

[2]PhD student in Animal Science by the Federal University of Minas Gerais – UFMG, Belo Horizonte, Minas Gerais, Brazil

[3]Adjunct Professor by the Department of Agricultural and Environmental Sciences of the State University of Santa Cruz (UESC), Ilhéus, Bahia, Brazil

ABSTRACT

Structurally, proteins are macromolecules composed of basic amino acid units linked by peptide bonds (amino group of an amino acid bound to the carboxyl group of another amino acid). In terms of nutrition, what distinguishes one protein from another is its amino acid intake. There are

---

[*] Email: veronicampb@gmail.com.

22 amino acids that form proteins, however, only 10 of them are considered nutritionally essential, which are among the nutrients that more impact animal performance.Therefore, it is of fundamental importance to know the food's amino acid composition, as well as its use by animals. Among the protein sources, soybean meal is an ingredient widely used in feed due to its balance of amino acids, on the other hand, like other plant foods, it has anti-nutritional factors that can affect the absorption and utilization of nutrients, especially in young animals.Animal byproducts can also be a good protein alternative with high digestibility, palatability and free of anti-nutritional factors.

Protein digestion begins in the stomach, where pepsin cleaves some peptide bonds. Like many other enzymes related to the digestion of proteins, pepsins are secreted as inactive precursors (proenzymes) and are activated in the gastrointestinal tube. The precursors of pepsin are called pepsinogen and are activated by gastric hydrochloric acid.

In poultry, food does not remain long in the proventriculus, passing quickly tothe ventriculus. At this stage of the digestive process the contractions of the wall grind the food, increasing its contact surface with the enzymes. However as well as in mammals, the protein digestion to polypeptides depends on factors such as the residence time of food in the proventriculus and the physical characteristic of the ingested protein.

To provide an adequate utilization of proteins from food, the first step is the degradation in the gastrointestinal tract (GIT) to the level of amino acids and small peptic chains so that absorption occurs.In order for this to happen, animals have a number of enzymes present in the digestive fluids which act in many different ways. Understanding this mechanism of digestion and enzyme activity in proteins in the GIT is important for defining protein digestibility of foods and therefore the biological value of protein.

The interest in researching appropriate protein recommendations for poultry and pigs has grown over the years due to factors such as increased protein sources' prices thus raising feed costs, greater availability of affordable industrial amino acid and limitation of nitrogen excretion predicted by environmental legislation.

Previously, diets for animals were formulated based on crude protein. In this concept, the amino acid amount was provided in excess or unbalanced resulting in nitrogen loss. Thus, the ideal protein concept emerged, which is to provide without excess or deficiency the amount of amino acids needed to meet the requirements for maintenance and production of the animal.

The ideal protein concept makes the diet economic by reducing waste of the second nutrient that most raises feed costs. Moreover it also prevents the additional energy expense to excrete amino acid that is supplied in excess, since it is not used by the animals as a source of protein. Finally, this prevents eliminated nutrient is released into the environment causing negative environmental pollution impact.

The ideal protein concept allows a decrease in protein levels provided once the proper level of limiting amino acids is maintained with industrial amino acids' supplementation in order not to impair the animal's performance. However, this requires formulating diets based on true digestible amino acids considering the relationship that exists between them, with lysine as reference.

Amino acids can be classified as essential, conditionally essential, and nonessential. Essential amino acids are those that animals can't produce a significant amount; conditionally essential are those that are, in a given situation, produced in insufficient quantities; and not essential are produced efficiently by animals. Essential amino acids are lysine, methionine, threonine, tryptophan, valine, leucine, isoleucine, phenylalanine, histidine and tyrosine.

The amino acids requirements for poultry and swine may vary due to several factors, such as nutrient levels, the animal's age, genetics and gender. Thus, many studies have been conducted to estimate protein and amino acid requirement considering these factors. Therefore, this chapter analyzes the main requirement recommendations of protein and amino acids for poultry and swine cited in the literature, as Rostagno et al., (2011), NRC (2012) and scientific papers published in leading scientific journals.

In this paper, sources, recommendation and protein metabolism in poultry and swine are discussed.

INTRODUCTION

Proteins are of fundamental importance in animal nutrition, as they are intimately related to the cell's vital processes and therefore, the body. Structurally, proteins are macromolecules composed of basic amino acid units linked by peptide bonds (amino group of an amino acid bound to the carboxyl group of another amino acid). From a nutritional point of view, what distinguishes one from another is its protein amino acid intake. There are 22 amino acids known that make up proteins, however, only 10 are considered to be nutritionally essential, which are among the nutrients that most impact animal performance. Therefore knowing the amino acid composition of foods is fundamental, as well as its use by animals.

Protein sources for monogastric animals can be classified into two categories: plant origin (including grain and bran as by-products of grains and vegetables' industrial processes) and animal origin (from animal tissues or by-products of the meat industry).

To attain adequate utilization of proteins contained in food, the first step is its degradation in the gastrointestinal tract (GIT) to the level of amino acids and small peptic chains, so that absorption can occur. For this, animals have a number of enzymes present in the digestive juices which act in many different ways. Understanding the mechanism of digestion and the enzymatic activity in proteins in the GIT is important for defining protein digestibility of foods and consequently the biological protein value. This paper addressed protein sources, its metabolism and recommendations on poultry and swine.

PROTEIN SOURCES FOR POULTRY AND SWINE

1. Vegetable Protein Concentrates

Soy

Soybean is a highly protein ingredient (35% to 38%), with large amount of oil (18%), fiber (15%) and other components such as sugars, water, etc. Soy protein has a high nutritional value because it contains all the essential amino acids being methionine and threonine limiting. Grains when processed result in quality bran, high in protein, which is essential for animal nutrition.

For non-ruminants, a thermally processed grain (industrial intensive production process) is important to neutralize their anti-nutritional factors such as trypsin inhibitors and chymotrypsin, allergenic factors (glycinin and b-conglycinin), lectins or soluble albumin and saponins.

Typically, these factors are eliminated by heat, however, one should monitor processing, since it can result in under-heating which would not eliminate the anti-nutritional factors or even in overheating, which promotes protein denaturation , or make them unavailable (Maillard reaction), damaging the amino acid profile. The most appropriate method to assess whether there was over toasting is the protein solubility in 0.2% KOH, calculated by the difference in percentage of crude protein on food and waste samples. This is a good quality indicator of protein *in vivo* (Parsons et al., 1991) because it quantifies the protein denaturation extent (by listing protein solubility in KOH and lysine availability). Ideal pattern of soluble protein in 0.2% KOH is above 80%, and below 75% shows sample super heating.

Urease activity determination (enzyme present in raw soy), through pH changes, is a method used to assess whether sub-toasting occurred, although it can not detect the soybean meal quality.

Protease inhibitors are protein compounds that complex with trypsin and chymotrypsin, impairing protein digestion already denatured by pepsin. The two major protease inhibitors present in soybeans are called Kunitz, with a direct trypsin specificity and greater sensitivity to thermal processing, and Bowman-Birk inhibitor capable of inhibiting both trypsin and chymotrypsin. Presence of these inhibitors leads to a reduced dietary protein digestibility due to the decrease in pancreatic enzyme levels that are free in the duodenum, stimulating more production of these enzymes by pancreas..

In young birds there is a pancreatic hypertrophic response when produced trypsin is not sufficient to neutralize the trypsin inhibitor, therefore decreasing protein intestinal digestion. However, in adult fowl, trypsin production appears to be sufficient in preventing proteolytic inhibition (Liener & Kakade, 1980).

Allergenic proteins in soybean are represented by conglycinin and β-conglycinin that cause hypersensitivity reactions in intestinal mucosa. Hypersensitivity reaction to soy proteins may cause changes in intestinal morphology, with villi shortening and increased crypt depth. Furthermore, conglicin and β-conglicin may be present in ileal digesta, due to difficulty in these proteins' hydrolysis, affecting performance of monogastric animals (Li et al., 1991).

Lectins are proteins found in most plants, particularly in pulses, and are often referred to as hemagglutinin, due to its ability in causing red blood cells agglutination in various animals species. They are capable of binding to specific carbohydrate located on cell surface, mostly cells of the duodenum and jejunum, damaging intestinal wall which reduces digestibility. Most lectins can resist digestive tract enzymatic action and bind to intestinal cells causing disruption and destruction of intestinal villi. This interferes with digestion and absorption of nutrients, reduces secretion of enzymes by enterocytes, causes hypersecretion of endogenous protein loss of plasma proteins into the intestinal lumen and increased mucous secretion from intestinal cells (Oliveira et al., 2000; Fasina et al., 2004).

Saponins are glycosides present in plants, which are characterized by a bitter taste, capable of foaming in aqueous solutions, cause hemolysis and complex with steroids, including those present in animal cells menbranes. Its antinutritional effects are related to changes in the intestinal mucosa permeability, inhibiting transport of nutrients and absorption of some compounds for which the bowel is normally impermeable.

Although the soy saponin level is generally low, fowl may be more sensitive than other monogastrics. Poultry fed diets containing 0.3% saponin presented reduction in growth rate, whereas the same level used in swine diets, produced no negative effect (Nunes et al.,2001).

Other factors, called flatulence, are associated with whole bean consumption, due to gas accumulation in intestinal tract caused by bacterial fermentation of oligosaccharides such as raffinose and stachyose.

In addition to these thermolabile factors, soy has non-starch polysaccharides (NSPs) and phytic acid that reduces its energy content and absorption of minerals such as zinc, calcium, iron and others, respectively.

NSPs, plant's cell wall main constituents, are sugar polymers that can not be digested by poultry and swine, due to its link nature, being resistant to hydrolysis in digestive tract. The mechanism of action is different between soluble and unsoluble NSPs, and they can be considered diluent nutrient or anti-nutritional factor according to their solubility. Water soluble polysaccharides act increasing intestinal viscosity by forming a barrier between enzyme, substrate and products of digestion (Classen & Bedford, 1991). On the other hand, NSPs' insoluble components can encapsulate nutrients because they maintain power generator nutrients inside their structures (carbohydrates, lipids and proteins) (Fireman & Fireman,1998).

An alternative to these polysaccharides is exogenous enzymes supplementation in animal feeds, such as xylanases and glucanases. Action of enzymes on NSPs probably does not provide great utilization of sugars by animals, but decreases viscosity of aqueous solutions in digesta and consequently increases nutrient utilization and energy from food. Simultaneously, a reduction in chain length affects the physical properties of NSPs, providing less binding capacity to other elements (Choct & Annison, 1992).

Phytic acid molecule, a phosphorylated myo-inositol, is an organic complex for storaging phosphor (P) in plants, corresponding to approximately 2/3 of total P present in plants. The higher the extent of myo-inositol phosphorylation, the greater is its nutrient complexing power, since the number of ionic charges affects its complexing ability, and phosphate groups deprotonation is closely related to the pH at which the molecule is (Oh et al., 2006).

Using commercial phytase in diets for pigs and poultry is a worldwide reality, sustained due to proven efficacy of these enzymes in releasing and making available phosphorus from phytic acid molecule and also preventing complexation of other minerals, amino acids and proteins.

Soybean Meal

Soybean meal is the most popular source of protein for poultry and swine, making it an ingredient that is strategically traded worldwide every year. Its protein rate is from 44% to 49% and contributes with 60% to 70% protein and 15% to 25% metabolizable energy in diets for broilers.

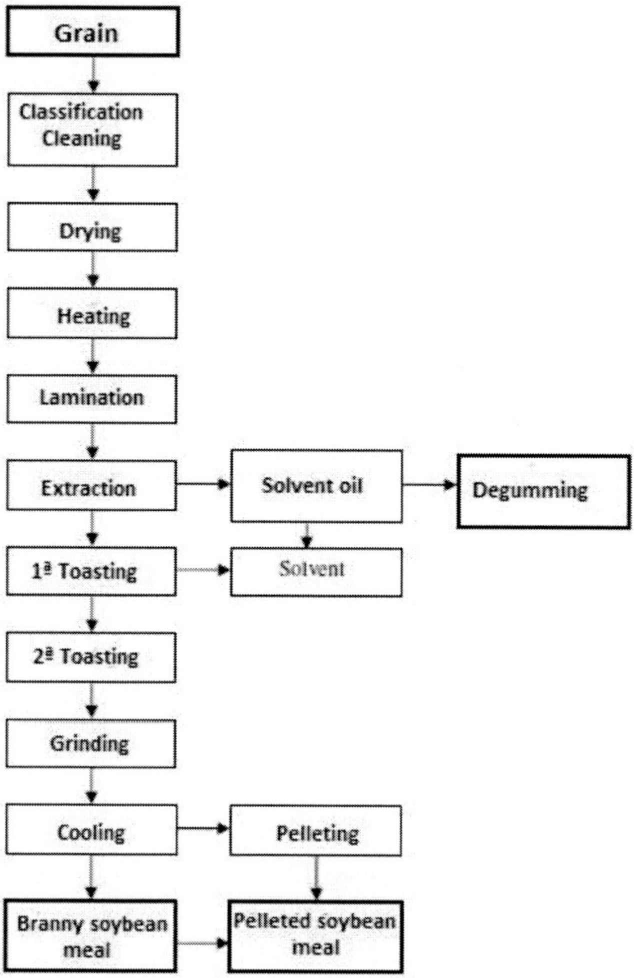

Figure 1. Processing of Soybean meal (Butolo, 2001).

The process for obtaining soybean meal (Figure 1) begins with the grains' reception, which undergo a sorting and cleaning process for removing impurities and, if necessary, they are subjected to drying, resulting in a product with maximum of 10% moisture and 0.5% impurities. Grains pass through a pre-heat treatment (620 ° C), followed by a mechanical process called lamination, in which are crushed to a maximum thickness of 3 mm. Later at the stage when there is oil withdrawal, when oil extractors of various kinds are used ("continuous" or "rotary" extractors). Here oil mixture extraction occurs with hexane solvent, which is separated and recovered from the mixture.

Extraction residual mass is subjected to two toasting chambers, which antinutritional factors present in the grain are eliminated by heat. In the first chamber is recovered a part of the solvent present in the dough, and on the second, drying occurs. After cooling and with reduced humidity, grinding occurs, turning soybean meal in mash form that will normally be packed in bags or be subjected to pelleting, originating bran pelleted soy.

Soy Protein Concentrate

After oil extraction, soya beans with pods undergo a process that partially removes carbohydrates. It can be used as an alternative source to milk protein, recommended for piglets as a partial substitute in the ration.

Extruded Soybean

Result of cooking soybeans by the extruder, with controlled temperature and under high pressure. Upon exiting the extruder, pressure is suddenly reduced causing immediate grain expansion. This is one of the most efficient processes for inactivation of anti-nutritional factors and improvement in nutrient digestibility because it causes cell wall disruption, provides greater exposure of nutrients, gelatinization of starch components, protein denaturation and shearing and restructuring of expanded products, dispensing product grinding (Zardo & De Lima, 1999).

Toasted Soybean

Grain cooking is performed by a heat source, with a temperature from 100 to 125 ° C and from 3 to 40 minutes depending on the heat source. Grain cell walls in this process are not broken and oil doesn't come into contact with air. Thefore, grains are not susceptible to rancidity during storage (Zardo & Lima, 1999).

Extruded Soy

Product obtained by heating (around 165 ° from 2 to 3 minutes), by direct steam, raw soy beans from infrared rays emitted through heated ceramic refractory, causing grains' heating from inside out. Subsequent to heating, shell is removed, and roller grinding (micronisation) is made until achieving the final particle size of 30 microns (Zardo & Lima, 1999).

This micronization process leaves the product with a slightly sweet flavor, making it attractive to piglets.

Canola Meal

Canola meal is obtained through canola seeds after its oil extraction for human consumption. Canola is a variety of rapeseed, an oilseed with a high percentage of erucic acid, very toxic for human and animal consumption. Canadian reasearchers genetically modified canola plant and evolved a variety with low acid content (Canadian Oil Low Acid - less than 2%). Canola meal has a nutritional value very close to soybean meal and can be a protein alternative source for pigs and poultry. It has less protein content (37.97%) and lysine (2.01%) and higher methionine + cystine content (1.64%) compared to soybean meal.

Despite the lack of toxicity, it should be avoided in starter diets for piglets due to its low acceptability, causing lower feed intake. To growing pigs it can be used in a proportion of up to 9% (Baidoo et al., 1987; Moreira et al., 1995; Zanotto et al., 2009) and termination, the inclusion up to 15% in diet doesn't cause losses in performance and in carcass (Baidoo et al., 1987; Gomes et al., 1998). However, other authors found that higher levels of canola meal in swine diets didn't have an effect on carcass' characteristics evaluated (Schöne et al., 2002; Roth-Maier et al., 2004; Thacker & Newkirk, 2005).

Summers et al., (1989) found no differences in weight gain and feed conversion in broilers with inclusion of 40% (100% replacement of soybean meal) canola meal in diet and supplementation with essential amino acids. Without lysine supplementation there was less weight gain of birds, evidencing that soybean meal can be replaced completely by canola meal, when supplemented properly.

However, Rostagno et al., (2011) recommended maximum inclusion of 3 and 5% in chicken feed in the initial phase and growth, respectively. For laying hens, recommendation is up to 4% rapeseed meal in the ration.

Peanut Meal

Peanut meal is obtained by mechanical means or pressing, or extraction of oil by solvents. There are two distinct types of bran: pie from shelled peanuts and resulting industrialization of whole pods, without peeling. The amount of peeling determines nutritional quality of peanut meal, and the peeled product has, on average, 48% protein and low fiber content (less than 15%).

Although it is a good quality protein food, peeled bran shows lower levels of lysine, tryptophan, threonine and sulfur amino acids when compared to soybean meal, thus it can be used associated with supplementation of industrial amino acids or other protein source.

Peanut meal has pleasant taste and smell, but it must be stored properly and for a short period of time to maintain these characteristics and not allow contamination by fungi, such as *Aspergillus flavus*, responsible for production of aflatoxins. Storage in low humidity environment, quick drying and careful harvest (peels and seeds undamaged) prevents fungal attack .

According to the NRC (1998), peanut meal has a crude protein content of 49.1% and 2,408 kcal / kg metabolizable energy for poultry.

Batal et al., (2005) studied seventeen commercially produced peanut meal and obtained the proximate nutritional composition and true metabolizable energy of samples. Crude protein values were found in the range of 40.1% to 50.9%, averaging 45.6%. Average substantial differences, in fat (2.47 ± 2.47) and fiber (8.3 ± 2.05) were observed between the samples, while ash (5.02 ± 0.59) was relatively constant and values of TMEn were substantially higher (2,664 kcal / kg) than reported by the NRC (1998). The total average composition of lysine, methionine, threonine and valine and their digestibility was 1.54%; 0.52%; 1.17%; 1.87% and 84.6%; 86.7%; 81.0%; 87.2%; respectively.

For laying hens, including this meal can cause minor redness on yolk color (Pesti et al., 2003).

For growing and finishing pigs, Li et al., (2000) suggest maximum level in the diet of up to 15%, considering that formulation is made based on digestible amino acids, so there is no decrease in weight gain.

Recommendation of Brazilian Tables for inclusion in diets for laying hens, broilers and to pigs in the early stages is up 5%, while in growing and finishing phases, up to 10% (Rostagno et al., 2011). However, use of peanut meal will depend on the availability and absence of mycotoxins, and costs.

Cottonseed Meal

It is a cotton byproduct, obtained from shelled seed after its oil extraction for human consumption. There are two products: cottonseed meal with 40% crude protein and 15% crude fiber (CF) and meal with about 30% and 25% CP and CF, respectively (Rostagno et al., 2011) (Table 1). The determining factor for this difference is the amount of bark and waste of oil refining.

Cottonseed meal can present clear golden yellow color (extracted by solvents), with lower oil content and less humid than the mechanically extracted, whose color can be dark brown, although it is dependent on the processing time and temperature.

Table 1. Chemical and energetic composition (crude material) from vegetables' protein ingredients for poultry and swine

	Cotton meal 30%	Cotton meal 40%	Peanut meal	Canola meal
Metabolizable energy for poultry (kcal/kg)	1666	1947	2253	1692
Digestible energy for swine (kcal/kg)	2222	2507	3475	3019
Protein (%)	29,98	39,21	47,77	37,97
Calcium (%)	0,23	0,87	0,17	0,56
Total phosphorum (%)	0,43	1,03	0,63	0,81
Phytic phosphorum (%)	0,50	0,59	0,42	0,54
NDF (%)[1]	42,33	29,40	15,6	24,48
ADF (%)[2]	31,11	17,00	10,88	2,05
Total lysine (%)	1,21	1,62	1,57	2,01
True digestible lysine (poultry)%	0,89	1,19	0,24	1,72
True digestible lysine (swine)%	0,71	1,04	0,26	1,54
Methionine (%)	0,44	0,59	0,52	0,78
Methionine+ Cystine (%)	0,93	1,27	1,11	1,64
Threonine (%)	0,94	1,34	1,26	1,57
Tryptophan (%)	0,51	0,51	0,58	0,49
Arginine (%)	3,41	4,43	5,31	2,32
Valine (%)	1,30	1,84	4,95	3,43
Isoleucine (%)	0,92	1,35	1,95	1,84
Leucine (%)	1,74	2,36	1,64	1,56
Histidine (%)	0,84	1,14	3,07	2,65
Phenylalanine (%)	1,64	2,20	1,12	1,01
Phenylalanine+ Tyrosine (%)	2,35	3,27	2,37	1,45
Glycine+ Serine (%)	2,46	3,57	4,18	2,36

[1]Neutral Detergent Fiber.[2]Acid Detergent Fiber.
Source: Rostagno et al. (2011).

Inside the seed there is a polyphenolic alkaloid with a yellowishand pinkish color element named "gossypol". Every gossypol in seed is free, non-toxic to ruminants, but during oil extraction processing part of the alkaloid binds to proteins (Prawirodigdo et al., 1997).

Gossypol complexed form is non-toxic to animals, because this complex is not absorbed in the gastrointestinal tract, however, a decrease in the availability of lysine and protein digestibility occurs (Ezekiel, 2002). Gossypol also complex with iron salts, which also fail to be absorbed (Chiba, 2001).

The amount of gossypol is variable depending on bran's cultivation and processing form. Oil extraction by solvents generates a product with less free gossypol and higher lysine digestibility (Phelps, 1966).

Experiments have shown that inclusion of up to 20% cottonseed meal, supplemented with synthetic lysine, does not affect performance (Henry et al., 2001; Gamboa et al., 2001) and carcass yield (Pimentel et al., 2007) in broilers. Ojewola et al., (2006) recommended the inclusion of up to 29% cottonseed meal in feed (subsitution of 100% soybean meal) with greater use of dry matter, nitrogen, ether extract and ash, and lower production cost, compared to lower levels .

In laying hens, gossypol generates a clear yolk discoloration, with olive aspect. However, inclusion of soluble salts of iron can reduce this effect by complexing with gossypol (Waldroup, 1981).

For pigs, Li et al., (2000) suggested maximum inclusion level of 8%, while Mello et. al. (2012) recommended the inclusion of up to 20% in growing and finishing phases without affecting performance.

In Brazilian tables, Rostagno et al., (2011) recommend for poultry and pigs inclusion 3-5% cottonseed meal in early stages and maximum of 8% in phases growth and fattening,.

Protein Co-Products of Corn

Corn Gluten Meal

Corn gluten meal (CGM) may be found typically with two levels of protein concentration, 21% and 60%. CGM 21 is a part of the outer membrane from corn grain remaining after extraction of most of the starch and gluten germ, by the process employed in starch or syrup manufacture through wet method.

After verifying the corn quality, classification is made including moisture, dirt, insects, etc. If the ingredient is approved, it goes a processing unit where it is macerated. This corn remains in the water for 35 hours below 50 ° C, in order not to gelatinize the starch and corn. Here the humidity is 40%. Next step is removal of this soaking water, which will go to a specific container, and corn is directed to grinding with three mills: the first, thicker, has the purpose germ removal, leaving it virtually integral; the second grind is intended to extract the remaining germ; and the third, thinner, releases starch from gluten and fiber.

Germ is separated and sent to press so removeing of moisture can happen (around 6%). Once dry, germ is directed to mechanical presses for oil extraction. During the grinding operation, after separating the seeds, the remaining product is washed in static screens, receiving a solution of water, starch, gluten and fiber. The solids (fibers) are retained and continue to presses and the remaining solution goes to the centrifuge, which will make the separation of starch and gluten. Fibers pass through the pre-drying and receive protein concentrate fluid, which is a water for maceration. Going through rotary dryers, with moisture of 45%, after drying, moisture is around 11%, generating the final product gluten 21.

Table 2. Chemical and energetic composition (dry matter) of corn gluten

	Corn gluten 21	Corn gluten 60
Dry matter (%)	90,00	90,00
Crude protein (%)	21,50	60,20
Metabolizable Energy (kcal/kg - Poultry)[1]	1750	3720
Metabolizable Energy (kcal/kg - Swine)	2605	3830
Digestible Energy (kcal/kg - Swine)	2990	4225
Total Calcium (%)	0,36	0,16
Total Phosphorum (%)	0,82	0,50
Neutral Detergent Fiber (%)	33,00	8,70
Acid Detergent Fiber (%)	10,70	4,60
Total Lysine (%)	0,63	1,02
Total Methionine (%)	0,35	1,43
Total Cystine (%)	0,46	1,09
Total Threonine (%)	0,74	2,08
Total Tryptophan (%)	0,07	0,31
Total Valine (%)	1,01	2,79

Source: NRC (1998); [1]NRC (1994).

Gluten and starch are left to be separated. Starch accounts for 70% factory production and, when separated in centrifuges, it goes to the finished products area as starch or modified, such as glucose or maltodextrin. Gluten goes to the dryer and after this process, it will have a moisture around 9%, being marketed as gluten 60. Gluten 21 shows high percentage of fiber in its composition and high content of total phosphorus, but low availability to monogastric animals. Its energy value is around 70-80% corn grain for pigs. Its low concentration of lysine and tryptophan, and low digestibility (Rodrigues et al., 2001) of essential amino acids limit its use, especially as a main source in these animals' diets (Table 2).

For pigs, corn gluten 21 can lead to a decrease in feed intake (Lassiter & Edwards, 1982; Cromwell et al., 1987; Trindade Neto et al., 1995), impairing the animals performance.

Corn gluten 60%, besides having a good protein and amino acid concentration, is a great natural pigment (290 and 0.12 mg / kg xanthophyll and lutein, respectively) (NRC, 1994), it is interesting to laying hens although it is also used in diets for broilers, pigs and pet line.

2. Animal Origin Meal (AOM)

Animal by-products are mainly a source of protein and minerals in pigs and poultry nutrition. Use of such slaughterhouse by-products reduces the diet cost, since these products replace partially or fully the expressive cost of some ingredients such as soybean meal and dicalcium phosphate. However, AOM have restrictions regarding its use because of its questionable sanitary quality and variability in nutrient composition. Both difficulties are associated with the control and processing of raw materials.

Knowledge of the material origin to be processed is essential to indicate the quality and, although routine analysis of each starting ingredient is difficult and due to its implement cost, it is necessary to pay attention to some quality AOM parameters, such as: bacterial contamination (*Salmonella, E. coli*), peroxidation of fats, presence of polyamines, possibility of *prions* presence causing spongiform encephalopathies, chemical composition, and amino acid digestibility of energy and sensory characteristics.

Fish Meal (FM)

Whole grain flour is the product obtained from whole fish and/or cuts from various not decomposed species, with or without oil extraction, dried and ground. Residual fish meal is obtained from cut and/or fish parts (head, tail, skin, viscera, fins) of several not decomposed species, with or without oil extraction, dried and ground. Ideal is having less than 10% moisture and NaCl indicated content (must be less than 3% and never exceeds 7%) in both fish meal.

It is an excellent source of unsaturated fatty acids, and also of good quality protein due to its lysine and methionine concentration, and is also a good source of calcium, phosphorus and other minerals. It is possible to find fishmeal with 54% and 61% crude protein (Rostagno et al., 2011). Energy value varies with the amount product's oil presence.

For piglets from three to eight weeks of age, the recommended content is up 4% in formulation and is not suitable for finishing pigs, even in small quantities, because of the residual fat fish that influences composition of pig fat, generating a thin bacon.

Maximum recommended is 7% and 5% for broilers and laying hens, respectively (Rostagno et al., 2011).

Blood Meal (BM)

Product obtained after heating the blood without coagulation, pressed to remove excess water, dried and milled. Conventional blood meal is produced from fresh blood without bristles, urine and digestive contents, except in amounts that can be admitted in good processing practices. The dark red product is insoluble in water and its strong scent may present an unpleasant taste or odor when used in large quantities in feed, above 4% (Miller, 1990; Cromwell, 1998; Fialho & Barbosa, 1999).

Blood meal can also be called flash dried or spray dried. Flash dried form is obtained by removing the water by mechanical process, or condensed by boiling to a semi-solid state. This semi-solid mass is transferred to a fast dryer to remove the remaining moisture.

This spray dried process generates dried blood by evaporation at low temperature under vacuum until it is approximately 30% solids. This mass passes in spray form using a device that runs hot air, which will reduce the moisture to a maximum of 8% and with 85% crude protein.

Blood Plasma (BP)

Product obtained from fresh whole blood, plasma spray dried (spray-drying), which was previously separated from its red cells by mechanical and chemical processes. Plasma contains a protein content above 90%, is rich in lysine and valine, however, with a low concentration of sulfur amino acids and isoleucine. It is low in calcium and phosphorus, but with high levels of readily absorbable iron.

Using plasma in piglets diets has a positive effect on animal development, immunity and intestinal mucosa (Van Dijk et al., 2001). This can be correlated with stimuli in feed intake, changes in the secretion of digestive enzymes, preserving the animals immunity and a lower incidence of diarrhea. Besides these factors, blood plasma could act as anti-stress factor by changing levels of ACTH (adrenocorticotrophic hormone) in piglets, providing better answers to the challenges, due to the stress of weaning (Gatnau & Zimmerman, 1994).

Red Blood Cells (Erythrocytes)

Made from clotting and centrifugation to remove blood plasma and subsequent drying of the erythrocytes, and it can be crushed. According Rostano et al., (2011), red blood cells crude protein content is 86%.

Hydrolyzed Feather Meal (HFM)

It refers to feathers clean and not decomposed, derived from slaughtered poultry, cooked under pressure and temperature. The presence of blood is acceptable once it doesn't significantly compromise the flour composition and, moreover, may be called "hydrolyzed feather meal and blood," when in high concentration. Feather is composed of keratin,

Keratins are rich in sulfur amino acids, particularly cystine, with values from 4.5 to 5.5%, and may reach levels of 60% digestibility (Butolo, 2002). The same author reports that due to keratin be extremely insoluble, feathers have to undergo a partial hydrolysis (acid or alkaline), so there is a partial degradation of keratin filaments, making it more soluble and more digestible, becoming thus, a good source of sulfur amino acid in the formulation of food. However, its limitation (3-6% in the diets of poultry and swine) is due to other amino acids, including methionine, lysine and histidine deficiency. Extreme temperature processing can still cause destruction of labile amino acids such as lysine.

Currently, researches have also been devised to promote the treatment of feather with enzyme mixtures containing keratinase enzyme, and results have shown significant improvement in the protein digestibility and hence, performance of birds.

Poultry Meal (PM)

It is the product resulting from cooking, pressing and grinding of poultry viscera, and inclusion of heads and feet is permitted. It should not contain feathers except those which can occur unintentionally, nor hatchery waste and other materials foreign to its composition, as well as being free from foreign materials and pathogenic microorganisms.

Hassanabadi et al., (2008) included 3; 6; 9; 12 and15% of viscera meal in poultry diets based on corn and soybean meal for poultry with 22 to 44 days of age and concluded that birds fed a diet formulated with 6% poultry viscera meal exhibited maximum gain and improved efficiency.

Silva (2009) using diets based on digestible amino acid (corrected for the same electrolyte balance) recommended inclusion of 5.3% based on the performance of birds. In the same study, the authors found that the inclusion of 12% poultry meal provided more abdominal fat.

Using poultry viscera meal in replacement of soybean meal in feed for growing and finishing pigs was verified by Pereira et al., (1994). Five levels of PM inclusion were used (0.0, 3.88, 7.75, 11.63 and 15.50%, corresponding, respectively to, 0.0, 25.0, 50.0, 75.0 and 100.0% replacement of PM by BM). The authors found that during growth, inclusion of PM caused reduced weight gain and feed conversion was worsened, although food intake was not affected. During the finishing phase, the level of inclusion of PM in the diet did not affect any of the performance's parameters.

Flour Hatchery

It is the product of cooking, drying and grinding the mixture of egg shells, infertile and unhatched eggs, nonviable and discarded chicks, fat removed or not by pressing.

Meat Meal (MM)

It is the byproduct resulting from slaughtered animals (cattle and pig) produced in slaughterhouses with tissue waste and carcasses condemned for human consumption, separated by dry, dehydrated and ground without bones. It should not contain hooves, horns, hair, stomach contents, blood and other foreign matter and pathogenic micro-organisms. Phosphorus level should not exceed 4% and have more than 55% crude protein.

Meat and Bone Meal (MBM)

It is produced in rendering plants and slaughterhouses with waste tissues and bones, after full boning the carcass of cattle, pigs or sheeps. This material is crushed, cooked, pressed to remove fat and is subsequently reground. It should not present hoofs, horns, hair, stomach contents, blood and other foreign matter. It must be at least 4% phosphorus and calcium should not exceed 2.2 times the phosphorus level.

When there is inclusion of cattle and/or sheep and/or pigs' carcass is called a mixed meat and bones meal.

Greater meat leftover inclusion than bone establishes the level of crude protein and macrominerals of meat and bone meal. The inclusion level is determined by the levels of calcium and phosphorus, which act as limiting, that is until reach the content indicated in the feed phase and the species in question.

The composition of flour varies depending on the species used, breeding area, animal feed, processing, etc (Table 3).

Table 3. Chemical composition of some animal origin meal

	HFM 75%	MBM 36%	MBM 55%	FM 61%	FVF	BM	BE	BP
Dry matter (%)	89,74	92,91	93,54	91,71	91,40	82,90	90,21	91,01
Crude Protein (%)	74,91	36,31	54,76	61,42	65,71	83,50	86,29	71,89
Calcium (%)	0,35	14,21	9,14	4,70	2,54	0,23	0,03	0,03
Phosphorum (%)	0,63	7,11	4,57	2,41	1,37	0,22	0,20	0,20
Fat (%)	6,13	12,63	11,54	5,85	14,63	0,46	0,51	1,09
Lysine (%)	2,32	1,69	2,91	4,33	2,84	7,55	8,62	6,54
Methionine (%)	0,66	0,46	0,77	1,61	0,89	1,04	1,22	0,88
Methionine +Cystine (%)	3,80	0,68	1,32	2,25	2,80	1,81	1,80	3,03
Threonine (%)	3,66	0,99	1,80	2,55	2,81	4,17	4,25	4,41
Tryptophan(%)	0,55	0,14	0,32	0,59	0,56	1,46	1,43	1,28
Arginine (%)	5,07	2,86	3,80	3,81	4,47	3,44	3,40	3,89
Glycine+Serine (%)	14,03	8,14	9,52	8,31	10,10	8,20	8,70	7,07
Valine (%)	5,56	1,32	2,46	3,04	3,86	7,35	8,20	4,90
Isoleucine (%)	3,56	0,80	1,60	2,49	2,82	0,69	0,49	2,26
Leucine (%)	6,47	1,73	3,16	4,40	4,98	10,97	12,40	6,99
Histidine (%)	1,07	0,51	0,99	1,32	1,18	5,09	6,03	2,16
Phenylalanine (%)	3,77	1,09	1,70	2,38	2,93	6,16	7,10	3,95
Phenylalanine+Tyrosine(%)	5,91	1,60	2,83	4,34	5,24	8,50	9,80	7,04

HFM: hydrolized feather meal; MBM 36%: meat and bone meal with 36% crude protein; FM 61%: fish meal with 61% crude protein; BM: blood meal; FVF: feather and viscera meal; BE: blood erythrocytes; BP: blood plasma.

Source: Rostagno et al., (2011).

Bone Calcined Meal

The bones of slaughterhouses are collected, crushed and burned. They are subsequently milled and packed. It must contain at least 15% phosphorus.

The chemical composition of some animal products used in feed for poultry and pigs are found in Table 3.

Digestion and Absorption of Proteins in Poultry and Swine

Protein is an important nutrient for poultry and pigs, being directly related to the animals' productive performance. Therefore, understanding the physiology of birds and pigs and specifically the activity of enzymes involved in protein digestion process, enables better matching of the diets and animals requirements.

According to Macari et al., (2002), plant origin proteins which are less digestible than animal protein, it happens because of the cell wall which complicates the enzymatic process on the plant cells content. Additionally, many factors can affect the digestibility of proteins, such as passage speed of food through the digestive tract.

The longer food is under enzymatic action, the more digestion will be increased in digestive tract. This can be achieved by increasing the amount of fat in food which reduces gastric movements, slowing the passage of food in the digestive tract, and hence improves digestibility of amino acids. Moreover, high content of fiber in the diet is associated with an increased passage rate of food through the gastrointestinal tract, which reduces enzymatic activity of the protein, consequently reducing the digestibility of amino acids.

The presence of non-starch polysaccharides also negatively affects feed ingredients digestibility, by increasing viscosity in the digestive tract, making the action of digestive enzymes more difficult. In this case, even reducing the passage rate, there is no improvement in digestibility.

Other anti-nutritional factors that hinder the digestion of proteins are inhibitors of trypsin and chymotrypsin present in raw soybeans. There are also phytates present in the vegetable ingredients, and that are capable of chelating nutrients positively charged and can form a complex with protein (impairing its digestibility) and proteolytic enzymes (inhibiting its activity).

Digestion of Proteins in Poultry and Swine

Digestion of proteins is initiated in the stomach, which pepsin makes cleavage of some peptide bonds by converting the majority of the proteins in proteases and peptones (Houssay, 1984). Like many of other enzymes related to digestion of proteins, pepsins are secreted in the form of inactive precursors (proenzymes) and are activated in the gastrointestinal tube. Precursors of pepsin are denominated pepsinogen and are activated by gastric hydrochloric acid (Ganong, 1993).

Pepsinogen (molecular weight of approximately 42500 D) is a non-active zymogen, because it has extra amino acids in its sequences, which prevents its action. It is activated at low pH (about 1.8 to 3.5), in the presence of hydrochloric acid, transformed to pepsin (molecular weight 35,000 D), or activated by other molecules of pepsin.

Pepsin can be classified in four different types: A, B, C and D having different actions in food's proteins. Pepsins A and D are secreted in the fundic gastric mucosa, while B and C are secreted in the pyloric mucosa (where the pH is lower). Regardless of the type of enzyme, its action is reduced at a pH above 3.6 and not occurring any action at pH above 6.0. Furthermore, it is relatively specific in its action on the substratum, hydrolyzing bonds between aromatic amino acids such as phenylalanine or tyrosine, and a second amino acid, so that the products of peptic digest are polypeptides of widely differing sizes. Also act on glutamic acid and cysteine or cystine, but on a smaller scale (Correia & Correia, 1985).

One of the important features of digestion by pepsin lies in its ability to digest collagen, an albuminoid which is little affected by other digestive enzymes. Collagen is a major constituent of connective tissue in animals and so that digestive enzymes in the digestive tract can penetrate the food of animal origin, it is necessary that the collagen fibers are first digested (Guyton & Hall, 2006).

During the acid hydrolysis in the stomach, glutamine is converted into glutamate and asparagine is converted to aspartate. As for the sulfur amino acids, cystine is converted to cysteine. There is also the possibility of oxygenation sulfhydryl groups of methionine and cysteine, cystic forming acid and methionine sulfate. Proline and hydroxyproline, which aren't α-amino acids, usually don't react during acid hydrolysis. Moreover, tryptophan, is essentially destroyed during acid hydrolysis. However, it is believed that the protein chain of tryptophan is kept intact (Nissen, 1991).

The digestive tract of poultry is shorter than that of mammals, being necessary a more efficient food crushing and protein denaturation in order to provide better digestion of proteins (Rutz, 2002). The food does not remain long in the proventriculus, passing quickly to the gizzard. At this stage of the digestive process, occurs food grinding, increasing its contact surface with the enzymes. However, as in mammals, digestion of proteins to polypeptides depends on some factors such as residence time of food in the proventriculus and physical characteristic of the ingested protein.

The proventriculus of birds is called glandular stomach, it secretes hydrochloric acid and pepsinogen (inactive precursor of pepsin) through the oxyntic glands, controlled by parasympathetic nerves. Hydrochloric acid and pepsin transform pepsinogen to pepsin (active form), the optimum pH for catalysis is low (acidic pH). According to Rutz (2002), the pH of gastric secretions is 2, but these secretions' dilution with digesta content promotes an increase in pH.

In general, only pepsin starts the process of protein digestion, accounting for only 10 to 20% digestion of proteins. This breakdown of proteins is a hydrolysis process which takes place in the peptide bonds between amino acids. As pepsins have optimum pH from 1.6 to 3.2, its action ends when the gastric contents is mixed with alkaline pancreatic juice in the duodenum and jejunum. The pH of intestinal contents in duodenal bulb is 2.0 to 4.0, but is about 6.5 for the remainder of the duodenum (Ganong, 1993).

According to these authors, pepsin is found at lower levels in piglets when compared to adult animals. At this stage, chymosin, a milk coagulating gastric enzyme, also known as renin is present in piglets' stomach in larger quantities (Ganong, 1993).

In the small intestine, polypeptides formed by digestion in the proventriculus of birds and stomach of pigs are further digested by potent pancreatic proteolytic enzymes and intestinal mucosa.

Proteases that act in this region can be divided into three groups: endopeptidases, exopeptidases and aminopeptidases. Endopeptidases and exopeptidases are secreted by the pancreas. Endopeptidases act on peptide bonds of proteolytic chains, whereas exopeptidases, also called carboxypeptidases, act on the carboxyl end portion of the chain, removing an amino acid residue. Aminopeptidase remove amino acid residues from the chain's amino end region (Longland, 1993).

Pancreas secretes inactive zymogens, which are activated in the intestinal lumen. The activation of pancreatic enzymes is initiated by enteropeptidase (formerly called enterokinase), synthesized by brush border cells of the intestinal mucosa. This enzyme activates trypsinogen to trypsin through removal of hexapeptide in proenzyme NH2-terminal region which, thereafter, trypsin does it self-activation from still existin trypsinogen in the gut, and other pancreatic enzymes. Enzymatic action of enterokinase has its optimum pH between 5.2 and 6.0. The major pancreatic proteolytic enzymes are trypsin, chymotrypsin, carboxypeptidases A and B and elastase.

Trypsin and chymotrypsin are endopeptidases that break peptide bonds at non terminal specific locations. Trypsin has three functions: auto-catalysis, protein digestion to peptides and chymotrypsinogen activation. To activate chymotrypsinogen, trypsin cuts a polypeptide from this molecule, transforming it into chymotrypsin (active).

Optimum pH for trypsin varies between 8.0 and 9.7, according to the substrate. Trypsin hydrolyzes only when the carbonyl group of the peptide bond is formed by lysine or by arginine and chymotrypsin hydrolyzes the peptide bonds formed by the aromatic amino acids phenylalanine and tyrosine. In general, trypsin and chymotrypsin transform large polypeptides into smaller chains.

Trypsin acts preferentially on already denatured proteins. For example, it has a weak action on ovalbumin, serum globulins, hemoglobin, collagen, etc. in natural state, but on the other hand, it digests them easily if they have been denatured by heat or other means.

Products formed by action of trypsin on proteins are proteases, polypeptides, peptones and some amino acids. It also differs from pepsin, which does not release amino acids in gastric digestion. However, some polypeptides don't disintegrate despite the action of trypsin (Houssay, 1984).

Carboxypeptidases are exopeptidases that hydrolyze bonds in the peptide carboxyl end, releasing free amino acids to be absorbed (Champe et al., 2006). Carboxypeptidase A hydrolyze aromatic C-terminal residues, while carboxypeptidase B hydrolyzes the C-terminal basic residues.

The main products of protease pancreatic hydrolysis are basic and neutral amino acids and oligopeptides, which are small peptides containing small mixtures of various amino acids. Oligopeptides containing six amino acids or less are more resistant to further hydrolysis by pancreatic enzymes and thus accumulate in the intestine lumen after a meal (Argenzio, 1996). Subsequent hydrolysis occurs in the brush border by enzymes secreted by enterocytes.

At this stage of the digestive process, oligopeptides are transformed into amino acids, dipeptides and oligopeptides in intestinal microvilli by the presence of exopeptidases which cleave repeatedly, the N-terminal residue of oligopeptides. Among them can be cited aminopeptidases and carboxypeptidases C and D. Oligopeptidases from the brush border are able to attack only small neutral peptides (Argenzio, 1996).

Amino Acid Absorption

For amino acids absorption there is a saturation kinetic, resulting in mediated transport. Amino acids in the L-isomer are absorbed more rapidly than those in D-form. D-isomers can only be used when converted into L-isomers (Lewis and Baker, 1995). This conversion or inversion consists of two steps (Baker, 1994): Oxidation of carbon alpha to the keto analogue; Transamination of the keto- analogue L-amino acid.

Conversion of D-isomer in L-isomer doesn't occur with all amino acids. Methionine is an amino acid which that conversion occurs. This makes that D-methionine bioavailable (Baker, 1994).

In poultry, a large amount of carriers are located in the ileum membrane, implying that this location has an increased absorption of amino acids. This, however, is not true for the ileum higher end, since most parts of the amino acid has already been absorbed. In pigs, as in other monogastrics, jejunum has a highest ability to absorb amino acids (Leibholz, 1998).

For poultry, at least three different amino acid transport systems, one for each type of amino acid, neutral, acid and basic. Moreover, there seems to be subsystems for neutral amino acids with a specific charger for glycine, methionine and other aliphatic amino acids, and a last for the remaining amino acids (Rutz, 2002). Acidic amino acids (glutamic and aspartic acid) has also dependent sodium transport systems and are considered less active in transporting neutral amino acids. Basic amino acids (lysine and arginine) have faster transport reactions to the interior of enterocytes.

The competition for transport proteins interferes with absoritvo process. For example, L-lysine absorption competes with L-arginine, L-histidine or L-phenylalanine, while L-leucine absorption competes with L-valine, L-isoleucine or L-methionine, (D' Mello, 2003). If amino acids are of L stereoisomer configuration and compete for the same carrier, inhibition may occur, which should prevail the one with greater chemical specificity, carrier affinity and concentration in the intestinal lumen.

The physical form in which a linker is associated to a binding site in poultry is quite broad, that is, onc amino acid may be carried by more than one integral protein membrane.

Di-and tripeptides are hydrolyzed to amino acids in the cytosol prior to entering the portal system (Champe et al., 2006). The absorption of oligopeptides of up to 6 amino acids and the absorption is more efficient and rapid when compared with the absorption of amino acids.

Low levels of vitamin B6 (pyridoxal), vitamin D, vitamin E and thiamine reduce the speed of amino acid transport. Another agent that inhibits the mitotic process and, consequently, the formation of enterocytes in the crypt, actinomycin D, also reduces the absorption of amino acids (Rutz, 2002). Any factor that affects intestinal health, impairs the absorption of amino acids.

The transport capacity of amino acids from the lumen into the enterocyte cytosol depends on the availability of carriers towards the substrate and the concentration of amino acids within and outside the cell. Thus, in the following feeding after dietary restriction (not severe), absorption capacity of amino acids is high because the number of available carriers is increased. However, if the restriction is too severe, a reduction in size of the villi, and the consequent loss (for peeling) of enterocytes (apical third of the villi) that has absorptive capacity may occur. In these circumstances, reintroduction of feeding has to be gradual to allow time to rebuild the absorptive mucosa (Rutz, 2002).

In piglets, the worst performance immediately after weaning is an industry concern and the main cause of this is the damage caused by reduction of food intake (Cera et al., 1988, Dunsford et al., 1989) which consequently will result in shortening of villi and deepening of the crypts leading to a decrease in the secretion of enzymes (maltase and isomaltase, sucrase and lactase) in enterocytes (Miller et al., 1984). Under these conditions, a higher number of cells produced in the crypts and fewer absorptive villi (Utiyama, 2006), impairing the absorption of nutrients by animals.

Protein and Amino Acid for Poultry and Swine and Its Recommendations

Crude Protein

Previously, nutritionists used to formulate diets for pigs and poultry using requirement values of crude protein (Araújo & Sobreira, 2008). Thus, amino acids supplied were higher or imbalanced with the animal requirement (Toledo et al., 2004), impairing their performance. In addition, excess amino acid supplied, besides making diets more expensive, contributed to environmental pollution, since its excess or imbalance is excreted in the environment, (Sá & Nogueira, 2009).

Amino acids supplied in excess are deaminated, being nitrogen converted to urea in pigs and to uric acid in poultry and excreted in the environment (Zanella et al., 2004). Thus, amino acid in excess also harms the animal performance as it is necessary to transform the nitrogen in urea (pigs) and uric acid (birds), diverting energy that would be used for animal growth.

So, seeking to improve the efficiency of amino acids utilization, diets based on total amino acids instead of using the concept of crude protein started being used (Araújo & Sobreira, 2008). However, when using requirement relative to total amino acids, it doesn't consider that a part is lost in the metabolic process, not matching the actual value of the animal demand. That led to formulating diets based on digestible amino acid values. Thus, it was considered that part of the amino acid that is provided in the diet is not absorbed, but is excreted by the animal. Although, as digestible amino acid, requirement values are most suitable, an amount of amino acids would be in excess, and therefore it was possible to observe a relationship between amino acids, therefore the ideal protein concept arose (Araújo & Sobreira, 2008).

Ideal Protein

The ideal protein concept is to provide the amount of amino acids, without excess or deficiency, which meets the animal requirement. Furthermore, there is the amino acid reference and all other amino acids will be determined according to it (Moura, 2004). The reference amino acid used is lysine, which was chosen because of certain factors like its metabolism (mostly for protein deposition), is usually the first limiting amino acid in diets of pigs and in second for poultry, easy to determine in laboratory, requirements of all the phases are available and economically viable (Araújo & Sobreira, 2008).

The ideal protein concept facilitated determination of amino acid requirement, because after determined the requirements for an amino acid, others can be obtained by the relationship between them (Tuitoek et al., 1997). Moreover, diet's crude protein content can be reduced without adversely affecting animal performance when supplemented with limiting essential amino acids. (Nørgaard & Fernández, 2009).

Reduction of crude protein and addition of industrial amino acids brought some benefits such as reducing the content of nitrogen excreted, and reducing energy loss used to convert nitrogen in urea and uric acid in pigs and poultry, respectively. It is estimated that a reduction of protein in 3 to 4% with industrial amino acid supplementation (usually lysine, methionine, threonine and tryptophan) has shown a reduction of 20 to 40% nitrogen excreted (USDA, 2003). In addition, less amount of nitrogen excreted reduces the amount of energy consumed, resulting in larger amount of energy available for tissue deposition, possibly leading to carcasses with higher fat content (Bellego et al., 2002). Moreover, crude protein reduction and amino acid addition can be excellent choices when animals are subjected to high temperature, because this protein has high caloric increase (heat generated in the metabolism). Bellego et al., (2002) working with reducing protein and adding amino acids in growing and finishing pigs observed no negative effect on performance, making them a good choice for conditions where the temperature is above thermal neutral.

Corzo et al., (2005) state that for efficiency in protein use, essential amino acids must be in quantities not exceeding those for optimal growth of poultry and a great level of non-essential amino acids is also required in order to ensure ideal ratio between essential: non-essential amino acids.

Lelis et al., (2008) evaluated the effect of diet formulated on the concept of ideal protein over nitrogen excretion and retention for broilers in the period of 1-46 days of age, and found that using ideal protein concept it reduced excretion and increased nitrogen retention, and can be used as a nutritional strategy to reduce environmental pollution.

Addition of industrial amino acids in the diet and crude protein reduction was possible by the availability of industrial amino acids such as L-lysine, DL-methionine, L-threonine, L-tryptophan and L-valine which allowed best balancing of feed (Sá & Nogueira, 2009).

Amino Acids

Amino acids are very important for animals as they are needed at all stages of life for maintenance, growth, reproduction and production (Nebraska and South Dakota, 2000). Amino acids can be classified as essential, conditionally essential, and nonessential.

Essential amino acids are those that animals cannot produce or they produce but in insufficient quantities to meet maximum growth of livestock and supply is needed in the diet. Essential amino acids for poultry and swine are lysine, methionine, threonine, tryptophan, valine, isoleucine, leucine, phenylalanine, histidine and arginine.

Non-essential amino acids are those that animals can produce in sufficient quantities by transferring amino groups (derived from other amino acids) to the carbon skeletons (derivatives of glucose and other amino acids).

And conditionally essential are those that animals under certain conditions, fail to produce sufficient quantities, such as poultry and pigs at the initial stage, weaning, or in sanitary challenge and therefore, there is the need of providing amino acids through diet. Perhaps, fixed-nutritional requirement determination for conditionally essential amino acids is difficult since it varies according to factors that influence their demand.

The following will be discussed on essential, non-essential and conditionally essential main amino acids, and its recommendations.

Essencial Amino Acids

Some grains are deficient in certain amino acids so grain combination allows more adequate supply of amino acids. As an example, combine corn and soybean meal. Maize protein is deficient in lysine and tryptophan, but shows high amounts of sulfur amino acids. Moreover, soy protein is rich in lysine, but has low levels of sulfur amino acids.

Limiting amino acid is one that presents in a lesser amount, being the first missing for protein synthesis. In main diets used for pigs, first limiting amino acid is lysine, methionine is second and threonine is third. As for poultry, the first limiting is methionine followed by lysine and threonine as second and third, respectively.

Lysine

Lysine is an important amino acid for pigs and poultry, first limiting amino acid in diets based on corn and soybean meal for pigs (Nunes et al., 2008) and second limiting for poultry. Corn contains 0.18% (pigs) and 0.19% (poultry) lysine; and soybean meal contains 2.54% (pigs) and 2.57% (poultry) lysine and HCl Lysine, industrial lysine, provides 77.5% (pigs) and 78.8% (poultry) digestible lysine (Rostagno et al., 2011).

Lysine is considered as standard amino acid in the ideal protein concept and has been used as a reference for updating needs of other amino acids. It was chosen mainly due to the fact that its metabolism is used almost exclusively to increase body protein.

Lysine is an essential amino acid and therefore is obliged to be provided in the feed, either by ingredients or by adding HCI Lysine, a source of very economical industrial lysine and therefore used in greater proportion in diets for pigs and poultry.

It has been noticed that lysine acting in maintaining integrity of the intestinal mucosa. He et al., (2013) evaluating the effect of lysine in weaned piglets, found that lysine is necessary to maintain gut mucosal integrity, particularly under conditions of stress, such as weaning. Also, lysine deficiency or diet with unbalanced amino acids or free of nitrogen can lead to increased expression of amino acid transporters, showing that deficiency of nutrients can activate the protection system of the body to maintain normal growth of animals.

Methionine

Methionine is the first limiting amino acid for poultry and second limiting amino acid for pigs fed diets based on corn and soybean meal. Corn and soybean meal contain, respectively, 0.29% (poultry and swine) and 1.16 (swine) and 1.13% (poultry) methionine + cystine, and DL-Methionine, an industrial methionine, provides 98.5% (swine) and 98.2% (poultry) methionine + cystine (Rostagno et al., 2011).

This amino acid is mainly used for muscle protein synthesis, however, it may perform other important functions, such as sulfur donor for compounds which present this mineral in their composition, as a donor of methyl groups in the organism and in biosynthesis of important components for growth and development of animals, such as creatine, carnitine, polyamines, epinephrine, choline and melatonin (Baker, 1991).

Furthermore, participates in synthesis of cystine by an irreversible process which has the function to remove excess methionine and overcome cystine deficiency. This is an important amino acid for protein synthesis, formation of skin, hair, feathers and production of glutathione (cellular antioxidant to the body).

Methionine + cystine is also used for animal maintenance, such as intestinal tissue *turnover* and therefore, its demand can be increased as the animal increases body weight and age.

Methionine can be added through DL-methionine, that is crystal clear, most economical and available, and hydroxy analogue DL-methionine in liquid form. These two sources are physically and chemically different (Ettle et al., 2010).

Piglets are able to differentiate and select appropriate levels of methionine in diet and sources of methionine. Roth et al., (2006) demonstrated that pigs were able to distinguish diet with different contents methionine and choose the diet with largest and most suitable content of methionine. Furthermore, Ettle et al., (2010) observed that piglets 21 days old are able to choose sources of methionine in evaluated diets containing DL-methionine and hydroxy analogue DL-methionine. They observed that diets supplemented with DL-Methionine were preferred by pigs over diets containing hydroxy analogue DL-methionine.

Threonine

Threonine is an essential amino acid that is added in the diet by inclusion of cereal grains, animal origin products or industrial threonine. Corn contains 0.26% (swine) and 0.27% (poultry) threonine; and soybean meal contains 1.55% (swine) and 1.57% (poultry) threonine (Rostagno et al., 2011). Industrial threonine is available as L-threonine, a source that still has high prices. L-threonine provides 96.1% and 94.9% threonine for poultry and swine, respectively (Rostagno et al., 2011).

Threonine is an amino acid that plays an important role in maintaining the intestinal barrier and intestinal mucosa against the action of pathogenic microorganisms (Mao et al., 2011) by production of mucin and glycoproteins.

Mucus, a digestive secretion, is mainly composed of water (95%) and mucin (5%) (Ajinomoto, 2003). Mucins are high molecular weight glycoproteins threonine-rich (Ajinomoto, 2003), which protect against intestinal injury (Mao et al., 2011). Additionally, antibodies are globular glycoproteins containing high levels of threonine (Ajinomoto, 2003). Therefore, in inflammatory processes threonine requirement by the intestinal wall can be increased (Remond et al., 2009). As the animals grow older, the need for maintenance increases, therefore amino acids involved in maintenance have their requirements increased, such as threonine.

Threonine plays an important role in the immune system of animals, a study of Mao et al., (2014), which evaluated three levels of threonine (0.74%, 0.89% and 1.11% which corresponds to 100%, 120% and 150% respectively of the NRC recommendation, 1998) in pigs weighing 5 to 10kg challenged or not by SPLV (attenuated Pseudorabies virus for pig). They observed that increasing threonine supplementation increased concentrations of IgG and IgM, and T-helper (Th1 / Th2) cytokines (related to normal immunity of pigs) and attenuated release of IFN-γ, IL-1β and TNF -α that were induced by SPLV injection. Moreover, they observed that increasing digestible threonine, it regulates TLRs (Toll-like receptor) 3, 7 and 9 expression in the tissue, relieving inflammatory responses caused by SPLV injection in weaned pigs.

Under immune challenge conditions, threonine can become the first limiting amino acid (Oliveira Júnior, 2012). Thus, it is important to adjust the supply of threonine because its deficiency can compromise digestive system functioning and immune system and reduce its availability for muscle protein synthesis.

The small intestine is mainly responsible for dietary threonine consumption. Thus, even if the diet is deficient in threonine, the small intestine has priority for using these amino acids and may compromise the availability to other tissues, as shown by Hamard et al., (2009), who conducted an experiment to evaluate protein metabolism by the small intestine, liver and carcass in weaned piglets at 7 days of age who received or not a threonine deficient diet. The authors observed that the protein metabolism by the small intestine was not affected when the animals received diet deficient in threonine, however, liver and carcass decreased the amino acid and protein content. Thus, it seems that the small intestine has priority by threonine over the liver and carcass when threonine is deficient.

Furthermore, in poultry, threonine with serine is present in important parts of feathers, corresponding to 20% of amino acid residues present in these structures (Kidd, 2000). It also plays an important role as a glycine precursor which is essential for synthesis of uric acid, nitrogen main route of elimination in these animals (Baker et al., 1972).

Tryptophan

Tryptophan is an essential amino acid for pigs, considered the fourth limiting amino acid in diets based on corn and soybean meal. Corn contains 0.04% (swine) and 0.05% (poultry) digestible tryptophan; and soybean meal contains 0.56% (swine) and 0.57% (poultry) digestible tryptophan (Rostagno et al., 2011). Tryptophan can also be added in diet by adding industrial tryptophan, L-tryptophan, that gives 98% digestible tryptophan (Rostagno et al., 2011).

Tryptophan plays important roles in protein synthesis, feed intake (Zhang et al., 2007), immune system (Le Floc'h & Seve, 2007) and welfare of animals (Liu et al., 2013). Melatonin (antioxidant), serotonin (neurotransmitter) and kynurenine are the major metabolites produced, and serotonin and kynurenine are the most important metabolic pathways (Lesniak et al., 2013).

Tryptophan can be used to improve animal behavior through production of serotonin, a metabolite responsible for the welfare of animals and reducing aggression (Liu et al., 2013). Post-weaning piglets suffer a lot with stress, and tryptophan supplementation is an alternative to reduce the aggressiveness of the animals and hence avoid losses in performance.

In addition, tryptophan can also be used as a stimulator of appetite. It works by stimulating production of ghrelin, hormone related with increased appetite. This was confirmed by Zhang et al., (2007), who showed that tryptophan increased plasma concentration of ghrelin and its expression in duodenum and stomach, and increased feed consumption in piglets. Ghrelin is a peptide released by stomach after stimulated by tryptophan. This peptide stimulates release of growth hormone and feed intake (Salfen et al., 2004).

Tryptophan also acts in the animals' immune system (Le Floc'h & Seve, 2007), with great importance when the animals are under stress condition, since this condition affects the immune system. Post-weaning piglets subjected to stress may have increased their demand for tryptophan because a part will be used for producing acute phase proteins. Thus, the ratio of digestible tryptophan/digestible lysine can be increased when the animals are under immune challenge and when a stimulation of the animals' appetite is needed. This ratio can also be altered due to environmental factors (Le Floc'h & Sève, 2007) or diet composition or second hand ingredient (Jansman et al., 2010).

Arginine (in Poultry)

Arginine is considered an essential amino acid for birds, especially in initial phase. Poultry have the highest requirement for arginine (Ball et al., 2007) due to lack of endogenous synthesis, besides the high rate of protein deposition by rapid growth of broiler inbred lines and antagonism with lysine.

Requirements for arginine in birds may vary depending on the growth rate and strain, and due to the fact that urea cycle won't be functional in birds (uricotelic species), they are dependent on the supply of this amino acid via the diet (Sung et al., 1991). Poultry cannot form citrulline from ornithine, because they lack the enzyme carbamyl phosphate synthetase.

Poultry also depend on additional arginine for formation of ornithine, which is in mammals obtained from glutamic acid. Synthesis of ornithine is essential, as is involved in getting proline, and is also used in formation of polyamines (spermidine, spermine and putrescine) molecules that are directly associated with growth and cellular differentiation.

According to Kidd (2005), arginine can go from fifth to third limiting amino acid in diets for birds subjected to high health challenge. Thus, it is believed that this amino acid may also be used for synthesis of proteins related to the immune system of animals. According Le Floc'h et al., (2004), this amino acid would be involved in stimulating DNA synthesis and cell division through synthesis of polyamines and increasing activity of macrophages by direct synthesis of nitric oxide.

Conditionally Essential Amino Acids

Glutamine

Glutamine is an amino acid that is endogenously produced mostly in skeletal muscle from glutamate and ammonia. However, under certain conditions, the demand for glutamine is greater than what animal is able to produce and supply it is necessary in the diet. Due to this fact, glutamine is considered a conditionally essential amino acid.

Glutamine is an important amino acid in cell metabolism and physiology. Glutamine supplementation in the diet, particularly in critical phases, such as post-weaning piglets and immune challenge, it can prevent intestinal atrophy, improve immune function and animal performance (Wu, 2008). Glutamine is required for synthesis of N-acetylglucosamine-6-phosphate, a common substrate for synthesis of glycoprotein, that is particularly rich in intestinal mucosal cells (Wang et al., 2007).

Glutamine is used as an energy source for immune cells and enterocytes, which are rapidly dividing cells. They are essential for synthesis of purine and pyrimidine nucleotides responsible for cell proliferation (Curi et al., 2005). They are also responsible for synthesis of polyamines by increasing expression of ornithine decarboxylase (Kandil et al., 1995). This compound acts by stimulating protein synthesis and deoxyribonucleic acid - DNA (Flynn et al., 2002).

Glutamine can increase activity of rapamycin target in mammalian (mTor), a kinase protein that regulates protein synthesis in animal tissue and cells, including skeletal muscle (Suryawan et al., 2006) and small intestine (Fumarola et al., 2005). Glutamine regulates synthesis of nitric oxide, a signaling molecule that regulates mTor activation (Pervin et al., 2007) and nutrient metabolism (Jobgen et al., 2006) in physiological concentration inside mammalian cells. It also plays an important role in synthesis of glutathione, an antioxidant most abundant in the small intestine (Wu et al., 2004).

Glutamine is an amino acid secreted in large quantities in the sow's milk and, therefore, very important to suckling piglets. This was confirmed by Wu et al., (2007), evaluating milk and colostrum within the first 28 days of lactation and found that glutamine concentration increases with advancing lactation and achieves a mean value of 3.5 mM at day 28, compared to 0.3 to 0.4 mM of glutamine in plasma of lactating sows. The largest amount observed may be explained by activity of glutamine synthetase in mammary gland and absence of glutaminase activity, contributing that glutamine produced is not oxidized in breast tissue and thus is excreted in colostrum and milk.

Arginine

Arginine is an essential amino acid for young animals, since its endogenous synthesis is not sufficient to meet the demand. Furthermore, the sow milk is deficient in arginine, which may increase need for addition in the diet (Maia et al., 2013).

Wu et al., (2007) observed that the level of arginine (free but linked to protein) in the sow milk until 28 days of lactation was lower than that of other amino acids such as glutamine with glutamate, proline, lysine and branched-chain amino acids. The explanation for this is that although the mammary gland has large amount of arginine, its release in the milk is reduced by some enzymes in the mammary gland (arginase type I and II) that break arginine, forming proline (O'Quinn et al., 2002). Thus, even though there is a greater production of arginine, a small portion is excreted in the colostrum and milk, on the other hand, proline is secreted into the milk since proline oxidase is not present in the mammary gland.

Dietary requirement for arginine, is high in young pigs due to its role as a carrier of nitrogen in tissue proteins and growth and gastrointestinal development (Hernandez et al., 2009). However, when the animal changes phase from breastfeeding to post-weaning, changes occurs in this requirement from essential amino acid to non-essential (Wu et al., 2007). This change is due to the increased concentration in plasma cortisol in post-weaning phase (Worsae & Schmidt, 1980). Thus, in larger animals, production of arginine, is sufficient to meet the animal requirement, therefore, in these animals arginine is not considered essential.

Thus, for older animals arginine is considered a conditionally essential amino acid because only in certain situations arginine production is not sufficient to meet the demand, such as in stress period. During this period, intestinal mucosal damage may occur and, thus, impair the metabolism of certain amino acids such as arginine, therefore provision is necessary in the diet for maintenance of arginine and reconstruction of the intestinal epithelium, enhancing growth (Hernandez et al., 2009).

Arginine plays important roles in addition to protein synthesis, as synthesis of polyamines, proline, creatine, agmatine and nitric oxide. It can also stimulate secretion of hormones such as insulin, growth hormone, glucagon and prolactin (Maia et al., 2013). Polyamines act by regulating DNA synthesis and protein synthesis and thus cell proliferation and differentiation (Igarashi & Kashiwagi, 2000). Nitric oxide plays an important role regulating blood flow from the placenta to the fetus, transferring nutrients and oxygen from mother to fetus (Bird et al., 2003).

Arginine can increase immunity of animals under immune challenge and to try to confirm this report, Mao et al., (2012) conducted an experiment to assess levels of arginine, (0, 0.5% and 1.0%) on concentration of betadefensina-procina (pBDs) in weaned pigs and found that arginine supplementation increases concentration of pBDs in some tissues and thus improves immune function of animals.

Hernandez et al., (2009) evaluating arginine supplementation in piglets observed that this amino acid helps in overcoming stress associated with weaning. Moreover, they observed a decrease in urea plasma levels when supplemented with arginine, indicating that this amino acid plays a metabolic role in newborn piglets.

Arginine may also improve litter size and fetal survival by elevating mechanisms of eNOS protein (endothelial nitric oxide synthesis), VEGF (vascular endothelial growth factor) and PlGF1 gene expression (placental growth factor I) in placenta surface veins (Wu et al., 2012). VEGF induces vasodilatation and facilitates the blood flow through the increase of nitric oxide.

Glycine (Poultry)

Glycine is a nonessential amino acid for birds, however, in initial phases, birds have a higher protein *turnover*, thus, rate of synthesis for this amino acid is not enough to meet its demand (Rostagno et al., 2003), being considered essential. In addition, diets based on corn and soybean meal with reduced protein level, can make glycine a limiting factor on animal performance (Corzo et al., 2004). Waterhouse & Scott (1961) demonstrated that the need of glycine decreases as the level of crude protein in the diet is increased.

Besides protein synthesis, glycine participates in the synthesis of purines and porphyrins (Shemin & Rittenberg, 1945), glutathione, creatine and uric acid (Christiman & Mosier, 1929).

Glycine molecule comprises uric acid, and, for each molecule of uric acid excreted a glycine molecule is eliminated. This fact has led researchers to believe that the requirement of glycine may be greater in fast growing poultry and in diets with excess protein or amino acid imbalance. Although this amino acid is synthesized by birds, this synthesis is not fast enough to meet the tissues needs and remove any excess of nitrogen, therefore, glycine should be supplemented in diet for poultry at an early stage.

Non-Essential Amino Acids

Nonessential amino acids as well as essential are also necessary for proper functioning, but may be synthesized *in vivo* from certain metabolites.

Cystine, serine and tyrosine are considered non-essential amino acids which are related with essential amino acids, respectively, methionine, phenylalanine and glycine. Methionine provided in diet can be converted to cystine, however, the opposite doesn't happen. So if a diet is deficient in cystine, part of methionine supplied will be used to meet the need of cystine. However, if cysteine is present in the diet, it reduces the amount of methionine required to be converted to cystine, thus saving this essential amino acid. Likewise, this also occurs with tyrosine and serine.

Antagonism between Amino Acids

Some amino acids may exhibit antagonism to each other. This happens because they display a similar structure that causes competition for the same place of transport and absorption in the small intestine. Thus, if an amino acid is supplied in excess, it can adversely affect transport and absorption of others, therefore resulting in deficiency of the other, even though this one is provided in adequate quantities (Nebraska & South Dakota, 2000).

Amino acids that can compete are lysine and arginine and valine, leucine and isoleucine. Main problems observed when antagonism occurs are lower feed intake, lower weight gain and worse efficiency gain (Nebraska & South Dakota, 2000).

Amino Acid Imbalance

Amino acids must be supplied in appropriate amounts so that the excess of one amino acid does not impair the metabolism of the amino acid that was supplied in adequate quantity.

Recommendations

By using the ideal protein concept one should pay special attention to the level of protein provided, so that it is not too reduced. Some studies show that the reduced protein to very low levels may change some amino acids into limiting. In general, supplying recommended levels of protein in the diet is sufficient to meet the requirements of arginine, valine, isoleucine, leucine, histidine and phenylalanine + tyrosine (Rostagno et al., 2011).

It is important to remember that protein retention decreases as the animal's body weight increases. Ringel & Susenbeth (2009) observed reduction in protein retention on average from 129 to 112 g/day when body weight increased from 35 to 135 kg when the same amount of lysine was ingested.

It is important to remember that the values of nutritional requirement may vary due to some factors that should be considered during feed formulation, such as genetics, gender, stage of development, feed intake, energy level of the ration, nutrient availability, temperature, humidity air, among other health challenge (Rostagno et al., 2011). In sanitary challenge, animals undergo changes in basal metabolism with increased energy expenditure and consequently reducing rate of tissue growth (Gandra, 2012).

Poultry

Broiler

Cella et al., (2009) evaluated diets with different digestible lysine levels while maintaining its relationship with amino acids methionine and cystine, threonine and tryptophan, for the performance of male broilers chicks from 1 to 21 days of age and set the value of 1.190%.

Oliveira et al., (2010) evaluated the effects of reduced levels of crude protein (CP) with supplementation of industrial amino acids on performance and carcass yield of broilers from 22 to 42 days of age maintained under heat stress, and it wasn't observed any effect of dietary crude protein levels on weight gain, feed intake and feed conversion of birds. However, reduced levels of dietary crude protein influenced the absolute carcass and chests' weights, which were higher at the level of 19.6% CP compared to 21.6%. Suggesting that the level of dietary crude protein using the ideal protein concept can be reduced from 21.6 to 17.6% in diet for broiler chickens subjected to heat stress.

Leeson (1995) stated that in broilers, as there is an increase in protein intake, due to the diet higher protein content, there is an increasing in breast yield, with a lower percentage of fat in meat.

According to Rostagno et al., (2011), protein requirements for broilers from superior performance in periods of 1-7 days, 8-21 days; 22 to 33 days, and 34 to 42 days of age are 22.40%; 21.20%; 19.80%, 18.40%; respectively. Aminoacidic demands for all phases of broiler with superior performance, according to Rostagno et al., 2011, are shown in Table 4.

Table 4. Exigências de aminoácidos de frangos de corte de desempenho superior

		Age (days)				
		1-7	8-21	22-23	34-42	43-46
		Digestible Amino acid				
Lysine	%	1,324	1,217	1,131	1,060	1,006
Methionine	%	0,516	0,475	0,452	0,424	0,402
Methionine+Cystine	%	0,953	0,876	0,826	0,774	0,734
Threonine	%	0,861	0,791	0,735	0,689	0,654
Tryptophan	%	0,225	0,207	0,204	0,191	0,181
Arginine	%	1,430	1,315	1,221	1,145	1,086
Glycine+Serine	%	1,946	1,789	1,515	1,420	1,348
Valine	%	1,020	0,937	0,882	0,827	0,785
Isoleucine	%	0,887	0,816	0,769	0,721	0,684
Leucine	%	1,417	1,303	1,221	1,145	1,086
Histidine	%	0,490	0,450	0,418	0,392	0,372
Phenylalanine	%	0,834	0,767	0,713	0,668	0,634
Phenylalanine+Tyrosine	%	1,523	1,400	1,301	1,219	1,157

Bernardino et al., (2011a) evaluated the effect of different digestible threonine: digestible lysine with or without glycine supplementation on performance of broiler chicks. And no significant difference was shown in different digestible threonine: lysine ratios on performance, however, it was found that supplementation of glycine provided better bird performance, demonstrating the essentiality of glycine for birds during 1-21 days of age. Furthermore, the addition of glycine lowered the activity of enzymes that catabolize threonine, enabling increases in the availability of threonine, thereby contributing to improve the performance of chicks (Bernardino et al.,; 2011b).

Tavernari et al., (2014) determined the optimal ratio for digestible methionine+cystine with digestible lysine for male broilers performance and Cobb females in two phases (11-21 days old and 22-35 days of age). The authors obtained methionine + cystine/digestible lysine ratios for maximum performance of broiler chickens, males and females, respectively, are 75.53 and 78.23%, during 11-21 days and 78.83 and 79.82% in the period from 22 to 35 days.

Laying Hens

For laying hens, proteins besides essential for body development also participate significantly in the composition of eggs. Leeson and Summers

(2001) described that the egg contains 12% crude protein, and 42% yolk, 55% albumen and 3% shell are proteins and these molecules have different aminoacidic profile.

Harms & Hussel (1993) comparing the performance of hy-line W-36 laying hens with 28 weeks of age that had undergone diets with 17.6% CP in diets of laying hens fed 14.8% CP with and without amino acid supplementation. They saw drop in egg production, weight and mass, as well as reduction in body weight of birds to diets with lower protein level and without amino acid supplementation. However, when the diet containing lower protein level was supplemented with amino acids that became limiting (lysine, methionine, threonine, tryptophan, valine and arginine,), there were no significant differences in performance when compared to diets with a higher protein level. In another study, at 42 weeks of age, the authors confirmed that protein reduction without amino acid supplementation harms performance of laying hens, and that supplementation with limiting amino acids in diets with lower protein level, the performance of the bird were recovered.

Rodrigueiro et al., (2008) estimated that lysine requirement for light-weight and semi-heavy reared from 4 to 6 weeks of age as 0.939% total lysine and 0.856% digestible lysine. But Filho et al., (2006) recommend a level of 0.92 or 0.84%, or 996 or 910 mg, total and digestible lysine/bird/day respectively for laying hens during peak production.

Matos et al., (2007) evaluated the influence of dietary levels of digestible lysine and threonine on egg quality of laying hens with 25 weeks of age and to improve eggs' quality, recommended levels of 0.70% digestible lysine and 0.50% dietary digestible threonine.

Sá et al., (2007) supplemented five levels of threonine in diets of light-weight and semi-heavy laying hens containing 14.0% CP from 34-50 weeks and found that threonine levels did not influence changes in body weight, feed intake, egg weight and internal egg quality in both strains. However, feed conversion, egg production, egg mass and Haugh unit were positively affected by threonine. And optimum ratio defined ideal threonine:lysine for light-weight and semi-heavy laying hens as 70.0% depending on estimated demands.

Silva et al., (2006) evaluated the effect of reducing dietary crude protein and supplementation of industrial amino acids on performance of laying hens in four periods of 28 days. They found that reducing dietary CP from 16.5 to 14.0% did not affect bird performance, but supplementation with lysine in diets with low protein content decreased egg production and mass and conversions by mass and a dozen eggs compared to the control diet (16.5% CP, 0.80% lysine and 0.70% methionine + cystine).

Swine

Pre–Inicial Phase

The post-weaning period is very critical for the animals once occurs dietary changes, going from liquid to solid food diet and ingredients with lower digestibility that affects the intestinal mucosa, impairing absorption of nutrients. This fact favors occurrence of intestinal disorders, which can happen more often when a diet with high protein content is provide.

In pre-initial stage, production of hydrochloric acid and protein that digests other proteins is smaller compared to adult animals and, as a consequence lower amounts of protein are digested. This greater amount of undigested protein promotes a growth of pathogens in the gut and a change of intestinal fluid and electrolyte balance, resulting in diarrhea (Nogueira, 2005). Therefore, industrial amino acids use is very common at this phase to reduce the level of protein provided. The major amino acids in diets for amino acids are L-lysine, DL-methionine, L-threonine and L-tryptophan.

Post-weaning piglets fed high protein level may be more predisposed to colibacillosis due to pathogens that ferment protein. Opapeju et al., (2009) assessing reduction of crude protein from 22.5% to 17.6% with supplementation of industrial amino acids in piglets at 17 days of age, observed reduction in proteolytic fermentation indicated by lower concentrations of ammonia nitrogen in the colonic digesta when animals received 17.6% CP supplemented with industrial amino acids. However, performance of pigs fed 17.6% CP and amino acid supplementation was lower than animals receiving 22.5% CP.

According to Rostagno et al., (2011), recommendations of crude protein for swine from 14 to 20 days of age, from 21 to 32 days of age and 33 to 42 days of age, are, respectively, 20.0; 20.0 and 21.0% and recommendations of digestible lysine for the same ages are, respectively, 1.520; 1.450 and 1.330%.

Nunes et al., (2008) evaluated the digestible lysine requirement (1.06, 1.16, 1.26, 1.36 and 1.46%) for males and females of high genetic potential from 6 to 15 kg (21 to 50 days age) in a thermoneutral environment and observed that the level of 1.46% digestible lysine gave best results of weight gain and protein deposition in the carcass.

According to Rostagno et al., (2011), recommendations of digestible threonine requirement for pigs from 14 to 20 days ages, from 21 to 32 days of age and 33 to 42 days of age are, respectively, 0.958, 0.914 and 0.838%. Digestible threonine /digestible lysine ratio for pigs from 14 to 42 days of age was 0.63.

Intestinal mucosa is the main barrier against pathogens and its integrity is directly related to the rate nutrients absorption. It is known that threonine is very important for maintenance of intestinal mucosa, thus about 50% of threonine in the diet is retained by intestinal mucosa of healthy piglets. Thus, knowing the importance of threonine to the intestinal mucosa, Wang et al., (2010) conducted an experiment in order to evaluate the effect of threonine levels (0.37, 074, 0.89 and 1.11% which corresponds to 50, 100, 120 and 150% of the NRC recommendation (1998) and threonine/lysine 0.311, 0.620, 0.750 and 0.930, respectively) on the intestinal morphology, and mucin production in epithelial mucosal barrier for weaned piglets. The authors found that the deficiency (0.37%) or excess (1.11%) of threonine negatively regulates intestinal mucin gene expression and results in a breakdown of the gut mucosal barrier (including villous atrophy, increased apoptosis and reduced mucin content). The highest level found to maintain the intestinal barrier was 0.89% of threonine, an important breakthrough in the prevention of diseases related to the intestine of weaned piglets.

Bisinoto et al., (2007) found threonine requirement and best digestible threonine / lysine for piglets from 6 to 11 kg of 0.72% and 0.49, respectively. Moreover, Zhang & Kim (2014) evaluating three digestible threonine/lysine (0.62, 0.67, 0.72) 0.62 noted that the ratio is sufficient for growth of weaned pigs.

Piglets from 28 to 56 days old were fed high levels of threonine (digestible threonine:lysine ratio) of 0.69 showed higher incidence of normal feces compared to the low level of threonine (digestible threonine:lysine ratio of 0.59) (Fernández & Strathe, 2009), which may indicate action of threonine on integrity of intestinal mucosa (Law et al., 2007). Moreover, digestible threonine/lysine of 0.69 tended to provide a higher weight gain and better feed conversion.

A possible explanation for different values found in literature may be due to differences in genotypes, levels of energy and protein and composition of raw materials in experimental diets, evaluation criteria used, ambient temperature, degree of activation of the system immune and levels of other limiting amino acids in feed (Bisinoto et al., 2007).

According to Rostagno et al., (2011), recommendations of methionine + cystine for pigs from 14 to 20 days of age, from 21 to 32 days of age and 33 to 42 days of age are, respectively, 0.851, 0.812, 0.745%. Methionine + cystine/lysine for pigs from 14 to 42 days of age was 0.56.

Recommendations of tryptophan for pigs from 14 to 20 days ages, from 21 to 32 days of age and 33 to 42 days of age are, respectively, 0.274; 0.261; 0.239%. Digestible tryptophan:lysine for pigs from 14 to 42 days of age was 0.18 (Rostagno et al., 2011).

Inicial Phase

In initial phase, animals are 15 to 30 kg and age of 41 to 64 days old. Recommendation of crude protein at this stage for barrows with high genetic potential for superior performance found by Rostagno et al., (2011) was 19.24%. The amount of digestible lysine requirement for barrows with high genetic potential for superior performance at this stage was 1.093% (Rostagno et al., 2011).

Oliveira et al., (2006) studied the requirement of digestible lysine (0.80, 0.90, 1.00, 1.10 and 1.20%) for barrows from 15 to 30kg, and found a digestible lysine level of 1.10 % for best performance. Moreover, Rossoni et al., (2009) evaluated digestible lysine requirement (0.88, 0.98, 1.08, 1.18 and 1.28%) for 15 to 30 kg gilts with high genetic potential and found a level of 1.08% digestible lysine for best performance results.

Recommendation of digestible threonine for barrows with high genetic potential with superior performance and digestible threonine:lysine ratio were, respectively, 0.689 and 0.63% (Rostagno et al., 2011.).

Saraiva et al., (2007a) studied the requirement of threonine (0.538, 0.577, 0.614, 0.651, and 0.688%) for females from 15 to 30 kg, in a thermoneutral environment and they found that the level of 0.62% of threonine (digestible threonine:lysine 0.67) gave the best performance for the animals. Furthermore, when assessing requirement of threonine (0.538, 0.577, 0.614, 0.651, and 0.688%) for females from 15 to 30 kg in high-temperature environment (32 ° C), Scott et al., (2006) found that the level of 0.587% threonine (digestible threonine:lysine ratio of 0.63) provided better feed conversion. These results show that thermal environments can influence the demand for amino acids by animals.

Amount of methionine+cystine to barrows with high genetic potential with superior performance found by Rostagno et al., (2011) were, respectively, 0.612%. and 0.56%

Moura et al., (2006) studied sulfur amino acids levels(0.502, 0.530, 0.558, 0.586, 0.614% methionine+cystine, corresponding todigestible methionine + cystine: lysine 0.54, 0.57, 0.60, 0.63 and 0.66) to castrated male pigs of high genetic potential from 15 to 30 kg, found levels of 0.582% and 0.588% methionine+cystine for respectively, better weight gain and better feed conversion, corresponding to a methionine + cystine / lysine ratio of 0.63.

Recommendation of digestible tryptophan for barrows with high genetic potential with superior performance and tryptophan: lysine ratio found by Rostagno et al., (2011) were, respectively, 0.197 and 0.180%. On the other hand, Fernandez & Strathe (2009) to test the relationships digestible tryptophan: lysine 0.16; 0.19 and 0.22 found better values of weight gain and feed conversion of 0.22.

Growth Phase

Growth phase may be divided between 30 and 50 kg and 50 to 70 kg which correspond to 65 to 87 and 88 to 107 days of age.

Recommendations of crude protein for barrows with high genetic potential with superior performance in two phases, found by Rostagno et al., (2011) were, respectively, 18.25 and 17.07%, and recommendations of digestible lysine were, respectively, 0.943 and 0.891% (Rostagno et al., 2011).

Abreu et al., (2007) evaluated the digestible lysine requirement (0.80, 0.90, 1.00 and 1.10%) for barrows from 30 to 60 kg and found the level of 1.10% digestible lysine for optimum feed conversion and deposition of lean meat. Haese et al., (2011) evaluated levels of digestible lysine (0.90, 1.00, 1.10 and 1.20%) for barrows from 60 to 100 days of age, they found that the level of 0.90% digestible lysine was sufficient to guarantee performance of the animals.

Gattás et al., (2012) evaluated requirement for lysine (0.65, 0.75, 0.85, 0.95, or 1.05% digestible lysine) for barrows from 60 to 100 days of age, found lysine levels of 0.96 and 0.92% for greater weight gain and feed conversion, respectively, and lysine levels of 0.89% and 0.90%, respectively, for carcass yield and amount of lean meat. Meanwhile, Serao et al., (2012) studying on levels of digestible lysine (0.83, 0.93, 1.03, 1.13 and 1.23%) met requirement value of 1.11% digestible lysine for females of high potential genetic from 30 to 60 kg to achieve best performance and daily rate of protein deposition.

Under heat stress conditions, requirement of amino acids can be changed. In order to prove this, Batista et al., (2011) evaluated the digestible lysine requirement (0.83, 0.93, 1.03, 1.13 or 1.23%) for growing pigs from 30 to 60 kg under heat stress conditions, 30°C and 34°C. The authors concluded that the digestible lysine requirement for animals subjected to 30°C was 1.05% for best weight gain and increased protein deposition in carcass, and environment at 34°C the level of 0.84% provided best weight gain and increased protein deposition in the carcass.

Recommendations of digestible threonine requirement for barrows with high genetic potential with superior performance in both phases, found by Rostagno et al., (2011) were, respectively, 0.613 and 0.579%. Digestible threonine: lysine ratio from 30 to 70 kg, is 0.65.

Amino acid requirement may change due to weather conditions and is important in determining values when animals are subjected to temperatures outside the thermoneutral zone. Thus, Saraiva et al., (2007b) working with requirement of threonine (0.50, 0.53, 0.56, 0.60 and 0.63%) for females from 30 to 60 kg, kept in thermoneutral environment, found that the threonine level of 0.52% (digestible threonine: lysine ratio of 0.63 gave best feed conversion).

Zhang et al., (2013) conducted an experiment evaluating different digestible threonine: lysine ratios for growing pigs (22-50 kg) seeking to obtain best digestible threonine:lysine ratio. In this experiment, the authors found that the best ratio depends on the variable response one want to obtain, so actual values was 0.70 for maximum daily gain, 0.68 and 0.63 for better feed conversion to minimize excretion of nitrogen.

Recommendations of methionine + cystine for barrows with high genetic potential with superior performance in both phases were, respectively, 0.556 and 0.526%. The methionine + cystine: lysine from 30 to 70 kg, is 0.59 (Rostagno et al., 2011).

Kiefer et al., (2005a) evaluated the methionine + cystine (0.448, 0.490, 0.531, 0.573 and 0.614% corresponding to methionine + cystine: lysine 0.54, 0.59, 0.64, 0.69 and 0 , 74) for barrows from 30 to 60kg in termoneuto environment (21.7 ° C) and found that the highest level of methionine + cystine was 0.549% (methionine + cystine: lysine 0.66).

Moreover, Kiefer et al., (2005b) estimated values of methionine + cystine (0.448, 0.490, 0.531, 0.573 and 0.615% corresponding to methionine + cystine: lysine ratio of 0.54, 0.59, 0.64, 0.69 and 0.74) for swine (30 to 60 kg) at high temperature (31 ° C) were 0.527% for maximum weight gain and 0.551% to lower feed conversion and maximum protein deposition in the carcass, which corresponds, respectively, the digestible methionine + cystine: lysine of 0.635 and 0.660.

Recommendations of digestible tryptophan for barrows with high genetic potential in both phases were, respectively, 0.170 and 0.160%. Digestible tryptophan: lysine from 30 to 70 kg, is 0.18 (Rostagno et al., 2011.).

Finishing Phase

Finishing phase can be divided into two phases, 70 to 100 kg and 100 kg to 120 kg corresponding to 108-133 days of age and 134 to 150 days old.

Recommendations of crude protein requirement for barrows with high genetic potential for superior performance from 70 to 100 kg (108 to 133 days old) and 100 to 120 kg (134-150 days old) found by Rostagno et al., (2011) were, respectively, 15.53% and 13.92%. Recommendations of digestible lysine for barrows with high genetic potential with superior performance for the same phases are, respectively, 0.829 and 0.748% (Rostagno et al., 2011).

Arouca et al., (2005) working with lysine levels (0.5, 0.6, 0.7, 0.8 and 0.9%) for barrows from 96 to 120kg, estimated that the optimum level of lysine was 0.610%. Moreover, Santos et al., (2011a) evaluated the digestible lysine requirement (0.540, 0.642, 0.744, 0.846 and 0.948%) for barrows from 95 to 125kg and found that levels of 0.803% and 0.817%, respectively, for better weight gain, meat deposition and feed conversion.

Recommendations of digestible threonine for barrows with high genetic potential for superior performance from 70 to 100 kg (108 to 133 days old) and 100 to 120 kg (134 to 150 days old) found by Rostagno et al., (2011) were, respectively, 0.555 and 0.501%. Digestible threonine: lysine ratio, from 70 to 120 kg, is 0.67.

Rossoni et al., (2008) evaluated threonine levels (0.480, 0.504, 0.528, 0.554 and 0.572%) for barrows with high genetic potential from 60 to 95 kg and found that 0.480% digestible threonine corresponding to digestible threonine:lysine of 0.60 was enough to get best performance and carcass characteristics.

Recommendations of methionine + cystine for barrows with high genetic potential for superior performance from 70 to 100 kg (108 to 133 days old) and 100 to 120 kg (134 to 150 days old) found by Rostagno et al., (2011) were, respectively, 0.497 and 0.449%. Digestible methionine + cystine: lysine, from 70 to 120 kg, is 0.60.

Santos et al., (2007) studied on digestible methionine + cystine (0.440, 0.464, 0.488, 0.512, 0.536% digestible methionine + cysteine), corresponding to methionine + digestible cystine: lysine (0.55, 0.58; 0.61, 0.64 and 0.67%, respectively) for barrows from 60 to 95 kg, they found that the amount of methionine+cystine was 0.507% corresponding to methionine + cystine / lysine of 0.63.

Santos et al., (2011b) evaluated methionine + digestible cystine (0.427, 0.466, 0.504 and 0.545% corresponding relations methionine + cystine: lysine, respectively, 0.57, 0.62, 0.67 and 0.73) for swine with high genetic potential from 95 to 125 kg, they found that the requirement that promoted greater meat deposition is 0.427%, which corresponds to methionine + cystine: lysine ratio of 0.57.

Recommendations of digestible tryptophan for barrows with high genetic potential for superior performance from 70 to 100 kg (108 to 133 days old) and 100 to 120 kg (134 to 150 days old) found by Rostagno et al., (2011) were, respectively, 0.149 and 0.135%. Digestible tryptophan: lysine ratio, from 70 to 120 kg, is 0.18.

Pregnancy

There is little research available on the demand for amino acids and their relation to pregnant and lactating sows due to complexity associated with fetal growth, breast growth, milk production and mobilization of maternal nutrient during pregnancy and lactation (Kim et al., 2009).

Feeding during pregnancy seeks maximum growth of fetal tissue and weight maintenance in order not to jeopardize the sow's reproductive performance in later phases.

In gestating sows, which feed consumption is restricted and supplied in one or two meals, one should be more careful when using industrial amino acids (Shannon & Alee, 2005) given that this metabolism is faster than in amino acids from intact protein, which can cause intermission between peak concentration of industrial amino acids and protein in the blood and thus protein synthesis is less efficient because for it to occur it is necessary that all amino acids are available in proper balance and simultaneously (Tuitoek et al., 1997). Thus, when using industrial amino acids a minimum of two meals are required so that an imbalance in the amount of amino acids supplied doesn't occur.

Requirements grams/day of crude protein for gilts from 0 to 70 and 70 to 114 days of gestation are respectively 300 and 360 and sows from 0 to 70 and 70 to 114 days of gestation are 285 and 354, respectively (Rostagno et al., 2011). Digestible lysine grams / day for gilts from 0 to 70 and 70 to 114 days of gestation are respectively 13.14 and 18.19 and sows from 0 to 70 and 70 to 114 days of gestation are, respectively 11, 18 and 16.36 (Rostagno et al., 2011).

Requirements of threonine grams/day for gilts of 0 to 70 and 70 to 114 days of gestation are, respectively, 9.70 and 13.46 and sows from 0 to 70 and 70 to 114 days of gestation are respectively 8.27 and 12.11 (Rostagno et al., 2011). Digestible threonine: lysine ratio for gestating sows are, according to Rostagno et al., (2011), 0.74.

Methionine + cystine grams / day for gilts from 0 to 70 and 70 to 114 days of gestation are, respectively, 7.23 and 10.00 and sows from 0 to 70 and 70 to 114 days of gestation are respectively 6 15 and 9.00 (Rostagno et al., 2011). The methionine plus cystine: lysine for sows in gestation are, according to Rostagno et al., (2011), 0.55.

Requirements grams/day of tryptophan gilts from 0 to 70 and 70 to 114 days of gestation are, respectively 2.50 and 3.46 and sows from 0 to 70 and 70 to 114 days of gestation are, respectively 2.12 and 3.11 (Rostagno et al., 2011). Digestible tryptophan: lysine for sows in gestation are, according to Rostagno et al., (2011), 0.19.

Lactation

During lactation, nutrition is important for better quantity and quality of milk production for litter, maintaining good body condition of sows so that it doesn't impair subsequent reproductive stages and reducing rate of disposal.

According to Rostagno et al., (2011), crude protein in g/day for lactating sows weighing 180 kg with litter gain of 2 kg / day is 897, weighing 220 kg with litter gaining 2.4 kg/day and 2.8 kg/day are respectively 1092 and 1280 and weighing 260 kg with litter gain of 2.8 is 1202.

Requirement of lysine in g/day for lactating sows weighing 180 kg with litter gain of 2 kg / day is 45.50, weighing 220 kg with litter gain of 2.4 kg / day and 2.8 kg / day are respectively 55.20 and 64.60 and weighing 260 kg with gain of 2.8 litter is 61.40 (Rostagno et al., 2011).

According to Rostagno et al., (2011), the requirement of threonine in g/day for lactating sows weighing 180 kg with litter gain of 2 kg / day is 29.12, weighing 220 kg with litter gain 2.4 kg/day and 2, 8 kg/day are respectively 35.33 and 41.34 and weighing 260 kg with litter gain of 2.8 is 39.30. Digestible threonine: lysine estimated is 0.64.

Oliveira et al., (2014) found that a threonine level of 0.608% and digestible threonine:lysine ratio of 64% meets productive and reproductive requirements of lactating sows with weight loss of 3.6% in average lactation period of 16 days.

Requirement for methionine+cystine in g/day for lactating sows weighing 180 kg with litter gain of 2 kg/day is 24.57, weighing 220 kg with litter gain of

2.4 kg/day and 2.8 kg/day are respectively 34.88 and 29,81 and with 260 kg litter gain of 2.8 is 33.16. Methionine + digestible cystine: lysine is estimated 0.54 (Rostagno et al., 2011).

According to Rostagno et al., (2011), requirement of digestible tryptophan in g/day for lactating sows weighing 180 kg with litter gain of 2 kg/day is 8.65, weighing 220 kg with litter gain of 2.4 kg/day and 2, 8 kg/day are, respectively 12.27 and 10,49 and with 260 kg litter gain of 2.8 is 11.67. Relationship digestible tryptophan:lysine estimated is 0.19 (Rostagno et al., 2011.).

References

Abreu, M.L.T.; Donzele, J.L.; Oliveira, R.F.M. et al., Níveis de lisina digestível em rações, utilizando-se o conceito de proteína ideal, para suínos machos castrados de alto potencial genético, dos 30 aos 60kg. *Revista Brasileira de Zootecnia*, v.36, n.1, p.62-67, 2007.

Ajinomoto – Boletim Técnico. Exigências de treonina para suínos.Benefícios da suplementação de L-treonina. 2003. Online. Avaiable: www.lisina.com.br, Acessc: 14 de julho de 2014.

Araújo, W.A.G.; Sobreira, G.F. Proteína ideal como estratégia nutricional na alimentação de suínos. *Revista Eletrônica Nutritime*, v.5, n.2, p.537-545, 2008.

Argenzio, R.A. Funções secretórias do trato gastrintestinal. In: Dukes, Fisiologia dos Animais Domésticos. 11ª ed. Ed. Guanabara-Koogan, Rio de Janeiro, 1996.

Arouca, C.L.C.; Fontes, D.O.; Veloso, J.A.F. et al., Exigências de lisina, com base no conceito de proteína ideal, para suínos machos castrados, dos 96 aos 120 kg, selecionados para eficiência de crescimento. *Arquivo Brasileiro de Medicina Veterinária e Zootecnia*, v.57, p.104-111, 2005.

Baidoo, S.K.; Aherne, F.X.; Mitaru, B.N. et al., Canola meal as a protein supplement for growing-finishing pigs. *Animal Feed Science Technology*, v.18, p.37-44, 1987.

Baker, D.H., Terrill, M.H., Kleiss, A.J. Nutritional evidence concerning formation of glycine from threonine in the chick. *Journal of Animal Science,* v.**34**, n.4, p. 582–586, 1972.

Baker, D.H. Partitioning of nutrients for growth and other metabolic functions. *Poultry Science*, v.70, n.8, p.1797-1805, 1991.

Baker, D.H. Utilization of precursors for L-amino acid. In: D' Mello, J.P.F. (ed). Amino acids in farm Animal Nutrition, CAB International, Wallingford, UK, pp.37-61, 1994.

Ball, R.O.; Urschel, K.L.; Pencharz, P.B. Nutritional consequences of interspecies differences in arginine and lysine metabolism. *Journal of Nutrition,* v.137, n.6, p.1626-1641, 2007.

Batal, A.; Dale, N.; Café, M. Nutrient Composition of Peanut Meal. *Journal Applied Poultry Research*, v.14, p.254–257, 2005.

Batista, R.M.; Oliveira, R.F.M.; Donzele, J.L. et al., Lisina digestível para suínos machos castrados de alta deposição de carne submetidos a estresse por calor dos 30 aos 60 kg. *Revista Brasileira de Zootecnia*, v.40, n.9, p.1925-1932, 2011.

Bellego, L.; Van Milgen, J.; Noblet, J. Effect of high temperature and low-protein diets on the performance of growing-finishing pigs. *Journal Animal Science, v.*80, p.691-701, 2002.

Bernardino, V.M.P.; Albino, L.F.; Rostagno, H.S. et al. Suplementação de glicina para pintos de corte submetidos a dietas com diferentes relações treonina: lisina digestíveis. *Revista Brasileira de Saúde e Produção Animal*, v.13, n.1, p.173-180, 2011a.

Bernardino, V.M.P; Albino, L.F.T.; Rostagno, H.S.; et al., Efeito de diferentes relações treonina:lisina digestíveis, suplementadas ou não com glicina, sobre a atividade enzimática em pintos de corte. *Revista Brasileira de Zootecnia,* v.40, n.12, p.2732-2738, 2011b.

Bird, I.M.; Zhang, L.B.; Magness, R.R. Possible mechanisms underlying pregnancy-induced changes in uterine artery endothelial function. *Journal* of *Cellular Physiology*, v.284, p.R245–R258, 2003.

Bisinoto, K.S.; Berto, D.A.; Caldara, F.R. et al., Relação treonina:lisina para leitões de 6 a 11kg de peso vivo em rações formuladas com base no conceito de proteína ideal. *Ciência Rural,* v.37, n.6, p.1740-1745, 2007.

Butolo, J.E. Utilização de ingredientes líquidos na alimentação animal. In: Simpósio Sobre Ingredientes na Alimentação Animal, Campinas. Anais... Campinas, p.295-305, 2001.

Butolo, J.E. Qualidade de ingredientes na alimentação animal. *Colégio Brasileiro de Nutrição Animal.* Campinas, SP, 430p., 2002.

Cella, P.S.; Murakami, A.E.; Franco, J.R.G. Níveis de lisina dogestível em dietas baseada no conceito de proteína ideal para frangos de corte na fase inicial. *Ciência Animal Brasileira*, v.10, n.1, p. 101-106, 2009.

Cera, K.R.; Mahan, D.C.; Cross, R.F. Effect of age, weaning and postweaning diet on small intestinal growth and jejunal morphology in ypung swine. *Journal of Animal Science*, v.66, p.574-584, 1988.

Champe, P.C., Harvey, R.A.; Ferrier, D.R. Bioquímica Ilustrada. 3ª Edição, p.534, 2006.

Chiba, L.I. Protein supplements. In: Swine Nutrition. 2nd ed. Lewis, A.J. and L.L. Southern, Eds.CNS Publishing. Boca Roton. Flórida. pp.803-837, 2001.

Choct, M.; Annison, G. The inhibition of nutrient digestion by wheat pentosans. *British Journal Nutrition*, v.67, p.123-132, 1992.

Christman, A.A.; Mosier, E.C. Purine metbalosm. II. The effect of the ingestion of glycine on the excretion of endogenous uric acid. *Journal of Biological Chemistry*, v.83, p.11-19, 1929.

Classen, H.L.; Bedford, M.R. The use of enzymes to improve the nutritive value of poultry feeds. In: HARESIGN, W.; COLE, D.J.A. (Ed.). Recent Advances in Animal Nutrition. Nottingham: UK, p.95-116, 1991.

Correia, A.A.D.; Correia, J.H.R.D. Bioquímica Animal. 2ª ed. Fundação Calouste Gulbenkian. Lisboa – Portugal, 1985.

Corzo, A.; Kidd, M.T.; Burnham, D.J. et al., Dietary glycine needs of broiler chicks. Poultry Science, v.83, n.8, p.1382-1384, 2004.

Cromwell, G.L., Stahly, T.S.; Randolph, J.H. Corn gluten feed in diets for growing-finishing swine. *Journal Animal Science*, v.65 (Supl. 1), p.39, 1987.

Cromwell, G.L. Feeding swine. In: Livestock Feeds and feeding, 4th ed., Kellems, R.O. and Church, D.C., Eds., Prentice-Hall, Upper Saddle River, 354, 1998.

Curi, R.; Lagranha, C.J.; Doi, S.Q. et al., Molecular mechanisms of glutamine action. *Journal of Cellular Physiology*, v.204, p.392–401, 2005.

D'mello, J.P.F. Amino Acids in Animal Nutrition. 2nd ed., 513p., 2003.

Dunsford, B.R.; Knabe, D.A.; Haensly, W.E. A comparison of dietary soybean meal on the microscopic anatonomy of the small intestine in the erarly-weaned pig. *Journal of Animal Science*, v.67, p.1855-1863, 1989.

Ettle, T.; Rademacher, M.; Htoo, J.K. et al., Dietary preference for methionine sources in weaned pigs. *Animal Feed Science and Technology*, v.155, p.201–205, 2010.

Ezekiel, J.M.B. Farelo de algodão como fonte alternativa de proteína alternativa de origem animal. Simpósio sobre Ingredientes na Alimentação Animal. Anais... Colégio Brasileiro de Nutrição Animal. Uberlândia. pp.137-162, 2002.

Fasina ,Y.O.; Garlich , J.D.; Classen, H.L. et al., Response of turkey poults to soybean lectin levels typically encountered in commercial diets. effect on growth and nutrient digestibility. *Poultry Science*, v.83, p.1559–1571, 2004.

Fernández, J.A.; Strathe, A. Dietary tryptophan and threonine supply to 28 days old weaned piglets. *Animal Feed Science and Technology,* v.154, p.265–270, 2009.

Fialho, E.T.; Barbosa, H.P. Alimentos alternativos para suínos. Lavras-MG, UFLA/FAEPE, 1999.

Filho, J.J.; Silva, J.H.V.; Silva, E.L. et al., Exigência de lisina para poedeiras semipesadas durante o pico de postura. *Revista Brasileira de Zootecnia*, v.35, n.4, p.1728-1734, 2006.

Fireman, F.A.T.; Fireman, A.K.A.T. Enzimas na alimentação de suínos. *Ciência Rural*, Santa Maria, v.28, p.173-178, 1998.

Flynn, N.E.; Meininger, C.J.; Haynes, T.E. et al., The metabolic basis of arginine nutrition and pharmacotherapy. *Biomedicine & Pharmacotherapy,* v.56, p.427–438, 2002.

Fumarola, C.; Lamonica, S.; Guidotti, G.G. Amino acid signaling through the mammalian target of rapamycin (mTOR) pathway: role of glutamine and of cell shrinkage. *Journal* of *Cellular Physiology,* v.204, p.155–165, 2005.

Gamboa, D.A.; Calhoun, M.C.; Kuhlmann, S.W. et al., Tissue distribution of gossypol enantiomers in broilers fed various cottonseed meals. *Poultry Science*, v.80, p.920-925, 2001.

Gandra, E.R.S. Relação lisina digestível: energia metabolizável em dietas para suínos dos 50 aos 100 kg de peso corporal. Tese (Doutoradoem MedicinaVeterinária), 67f.UNESP-Botucatu, 2012.

Ganong, W.F. Fisiologia Médica. 15ª ed. Prentice-Hall do Brasil, 1993.

Gatnau, R.; Zimmerman, D.R. Effects spray dried plasma of different sources and process on growth performance of weanling pigs. *Journal of Animal Science*, v.72: p.166, 1994 (Suppl. 1).

Gattás, G.; Silva, F.C.O.; Barbosa, F.F. et al., Níveis de lisina digestível em dietas para suínos machos castrados dos 60 aos 100 dias de idade. *Revista Brasileira de Zootecnia*, v.41, n.1, p.91-97, 2012.

Gomes, P.C.; Zanotto, D.L.; Guidoni, A.L. et al., Uso do farelo de canola para suínos na fase de terminação. *Revista Brasileira de Zootecnia*, v.27, p.749-753, 1998.

Guyton, A.C.; Hall, J.E. Tratado de Fisiologia Médica. 11ª ed.; Ed. Guanabara-Koogan; 2006.

Haese, D.; Donzele, J.L.; Oliveira, R.F.M. et al., Digestible lysine for barrows of genetic lines selected for meat deposition from 60 to 100 days of age. *Revista Brasileira de Zootecnia*, v.40, n.9, p.1941-1946, 2011.

Hamard, A.; Sève, B.; Le Floc'h, N. A moderate threonine deficiency differently affects protein metabolism in tissues of early-weaned piglets. *Comparative Biochemistry and Physiology*, v.52, p.491–497, 2009.

Harms, R.H.; Russel, G.B. Optimizing egg mass with amino acid supplementation of a low protein diet. *Poultry Science*, v.72, n.1, p.1892-1896, 1993.

Hassanabadi, A.; Amanloo, H.; Zamanian, M. Effects of substitution of soybean meal with poultry by-product meal on broiler chickens performance. *Journal of Animal and Veterinary Advances*, v.7, p.303-307, 2008.

He, L.; Yang, H.; Hou, Y. et al., Effects of dietary L-lysine intake on the intestinal mucosa and expression of CAT genes in weaned piglets. *Amino Acids,* v.45, p.383–391, 2013.

Heny, M.H.; Pesti, G.M.; Bakalli, R. et al., The performance or broiler chicks fed diets containing extruded cottonseed meal supplemented with lysine. *Poultry Science,* v.80, p.762-8, 2001.

Hernandez, A.; Hansen, C.F.; Mullan, B.P. et al., l-arginine supplementation of milk liquid or dry diets fed to pigs after weaning has a positive effect on production in the first three weeks after weaning at 21 days of age. *Animal Feed Science and Technology*, v.154, p.102–111, 2009.

Houssay, B.A. Fisiologia Humana. 5[a] ed., Guanabara Koogan, p.273-303, 1984.

Igarashi, K.; Kashiwagi, K. Polyamines: mysterious modulators of cellular functions. *Biochemical and Biophysical Research Communications*, v.271, p.559–564, 2000.

Jansman, A.J.M.; Van Diepen, J.TH.M.; Melchior, D. The effect of diet composition on tryptophan requirement of young piglets. *Journal Animal Science*, v.88, p.1017-1027, 2010.

Jobgen, W.S.; Fried, S.K.; Fu, W.J. et al., Regulatory role for the arginine-nitric oxide pathway in metabolism of energy substrates. *Journal Nutrition Biochemistry,* v.17, p.571–588, 2006.

Kandil, H.M.; Argenzio, R.A.; Chen, W. et al., L-Glutamine and L-asparagine stimulate ODC activity and proliferation in a porcine jejunal enterocytes line. *American Journal of Physiology*, v.269, p.G591–G599, 1995.

Kidd, M.T. Nutritional considerations concerning threonine in broiles. *World's Poultry Science Journal*, v.56, n.2, p.139-151, 2000.

Kidd, M.T. Relationship between the nutritional requirements and the immune system in poultry. 2 SIMPOSIO INTERNACIONAL SOBRE EXIGENCIAS NUTRICIONAIS DE AVES E SUÍNOS. 2005: Viçosa:MG. Anais... Viçosa:UFV, p.61-73, 2005.

Kiefer, C.; Ferreira, A.S.; Donzele, J.L. et al., Exigência de metionina + cistina digestíveis para suínos mantidos em ambiente termoneutro dos 30 aos 60 kg. *Revista Brasileira de Zootecnia*, v.34, n.3, p.847-854, 2005a.

Kiefer, C.; Ferreira, A.S.; Oliveira, R.F.M. et al., Exigência de metionina mais cistina digestíveis para suínos machos castrados mantidos em ambiente de alta temperatura dos 30 aos 60 kg. *Revista Brasileira de Zootecnia*, v.34, n.1, p.104-111, 2005b.

Kim, S.W.; Hurley, W.L.; Wu, G. et al., Ideal amino acid balance for sows during gestation and lactation1. *Journal Animal Science*, v.87, p.E123-E132, 2009.

Lassiter, J.W.; Edwards Jr.; H.M. Animal nutrition. Virginia: Reston Publishing Company, p.339-340, 1982.

Law, G.K.; Bertolo, F.P.; Adjiri-Awere, A. et al., Adequate oral THR is critical for mucin production and gut function in neonatal piglets. *American Journal* of *Physiology - Gastrointestinal* and *Liver Physiology*, v.292, p.G1293–G1301, 2007.

Leeson, S. Nutrição e qualidade da carcaça de frangos de corte. In: CONFERÊNCIA APINCO, 1995, Campinas. Simpósio Internacional Sobre Ambiência e Instalações na Avicultura Industrial. Anais... Campinas: Fundação Apinco de Ciência e Tecnologia Avícola. p.111-118, 1995.

Leeson, S.; Summers, J.D. Nutrition of the chicken. 4th edition, 591p., 2001.

Le Floc'H, N.; Melchior, D.; Obled, C. Modifications of protein and amino acid metabolism during inflamation and immune system activation. *Livestock Production Science*, v.87, p.37-45, 2004.

Le Floc'h, N.; Seve, B. Biological roles of tryptophan and its metabolism: Potential implications for pig feeding. *Livestock Science*, v.112, p.23–32, 2007.

Lelis. G.R.; Lora, A.G.; Albino, L.F.T. et al., Influência da dieta formulada no conceito de proteína ideal sobre a excreção e a retenção de nitrogênio em frangos de corte. In: CONFERÊNCIA APINCO, 2008, *Santos. Anais...* p.153, 2008.

Lesniak, W.G.; Jyoti, A.; Mishra, M.K. et al., Concurrent quantification of tryptophan and its major metabolites. *Analytical Biochemistry*, v.443, p.222–231, 2013.

Lewis, A.J.; Baker, D.H. Bioaavailability of D- Amino Acids and DL-Hydroxy Methionine. In: *Bioaavailability of Nutrients for Animals*. Academic Press. Ammermam et all. 1995.

Li, D.F.; Nelssen, J.L.; Reddy, P.G.; Blecha, F.; Klemm, R.D.; Giesting, D.W.; Hancock, J.D.; Allee, G.L.; Goodband, R.D. Measuring suitability of soybean products for early-weaned pigs with immunological criteria. *Journal of Animal Science*, v.69, p.3299-3307, 1991.

Li, D.F.; Xu, X.X.; Qiao, S.Y. Growth performance of growing-finishing pigs fed diets supplemented with Chinese cottonseed meal based on amino acids digestibilities. *Asian-Australasian Journal of Animal Sciences*, v.13, p.521-527, 2000.

Liener, I.E.; Kakade, M.L. Protease inhibitors. In: Toxic constituentes of plant foodstuffs, 2nd ed. I.E. Liener, ed. Acadmic press: New York., 1980.

Liu, H.; Shi, B.M.; Shan, A.S. Supplemental dietary tryptophan modifies behavior, concentrations of salivary cortisol, plasma epinephrine, norepinephrine and hypothalamic 5-hydroxytryptaminein weaning piglets. *Livestock Science*, v.151, p.213–218, 2013.

Longland, A.C. In Vitro Digestion for Pigs and Poultry. Ed. M.F. Fuller, 1991.

Macari, M.; Furlan, R.L.; Gonzáles, E. Fisiologia *Aviária Aplicada a Frangos de Corte*. 2ª ed. FUNEP, 2002.

Maia, R.C.; Silva, A.D.; Albino, L.F.T. Funções imunológicas dos aminoácidos para suínos. *Revista Eletrônica de Pesquisa Animal*, v.01, n.02, p.137-156, 2013.

Mao, X.; Lai, X.; Yu, B. et al., Effects of dietary threonine supplementation on immune challenge induced by swine Pseudorabies live vaccine in weaned pigs. *Archives of Animal Nutrition*, v.68, n.1, p.1–15, 2014.

Mao, X.; Qi, S.; Yu, B. rt al., D. Dietary L-arginine supplementation enhances porcine b-defensins gene expression in some tissues of weaned pigs. *Livestock Science*, v.148, p.103–108, 2012.

Mao, X.; Zeng, X.; Qiao, S. et al., Specific roles of threonine in intestinal mucosal integrity and barrier function. *Frontiers of Bioscience*, v.3, p.1192-1200, 2011.

Matos, M.S.; Leandro, N.S.M.; Carvalho, F.B. et al., Qualidade interna e externa de ovos de poedeiras comerciais alimentadas com rações contendo níveis de lisina e treonina digestível. In: CONFERÊNCIA APINCO, 2007, *Santos. Anais*... p.154, 2007.

Mello, G.; Laurentiz, A.C.; Filardi, R.S. et al., Farelo de algodão em rações para suínos nas fases de crescimento e terminação. *Archivos de Zootecnia,* v.61, p.55-62, 2012.

Miler, E.D. Blood-meal: flash-dried. In: Nontraditional Feed Sources for Use in Swine Production. Tacker, P.A., and Kirkwood, R.N., Eds., Butterworths, Boston, 1990.

Miller, B.G.;Newby, T.J.; Stokes, C.R. et al., Influence of diet on postweaning malabsortion and diarrhoea in the pig. *Research in Veterinary Science,* v.36. p.187-193, 1984.

Moreira, I.; Furlan, A.C.; Scapinello, C. et al., Utilização do farelo de canola na alimentação de suínos na fase inicial (42 a 63 dias). *Revista Brasileira de Zootecnia*, v.24, p.417-427, 1995.

Moura, A.M.A. Conceito da proteína ideal aplicada na nutrição de aves e suínos. *Revista Eletrônica Nutritime*, v.1, n.1, p.31-34, 2004.

Moura, J.O.; Brustolini, P.C.; Silva, F.C.O. et al., Exigências de aminoácidos sulfurados digestíveis para suínos machos castrados e fêmeas de 15 a 30 kg. *Revista Brasileira de Zootecnia*, v.35, n.3, p.1085-1090, 2006 (supl.).

Nebraska and South Dakota. 2000. Swine Nutrition Guide. Livro. 44p. This publication is available at: http://ianrwww.unl.edu/pubs/swine/ec273.htm.

Nissen, S. Modem Methods in Protein Nutrition and Metabolism. Academic Press., 1991.

NRC. National Research Council. *Nutrient Requeriments of Poultry.* Washington. 155p., 1994.

Nogueira, E.T. Aminoácidos: essenciais para Suínos. Suinocultura Industrial, Edição 191, v.08, p.26 - 28. 2005.

Nørgaard, J.V.; Fernández, J.A. Isoleucine and valine supplementation of crude protein-reduced diets for pigs aged 5–8 weeks. *Animal Feed Science and Technology*, v.154, p.248–253, 2009.

NRC. National Research Council.Nutrient requirements of swine. 10ª ed. National Academy of Science.Washington, D.C. 189 pp., 1998.

Nunes, R.V. Fatores antinutricionais dos ingredientes destinados à alimentação animal. In: SIMPÓSIO SOBRE INGREDIENTES NA ALIMENTAÇÃO ANIMAL, 2001, Campinas. Anais... Campinas: CBNA, p.235-266, 2001.

Nunes, C.G.V.; Oliveira, R.F.M.; Donzele, J.L. et al., Níveis de lisina digestível para leitões dos 6 aos 15 kg. *Revista Brasileira de Zootecnia,* v.37, n.1, p.84-88, 2008.

Oh, B.C.; Kim, M.H.; Yun, B.S. et al., Ca^{+2}- inositol phosphate checation mediates the substrate specificity of β-propeller phytase. *Biochemistry,* v.45, p.9531-9539, 2006.

Ojewola, G.S.; Ukachukwu, S.N.; Okulonye, E.I. Cottonseed Meal as Substitute for Soyabean Meal in Broiler Ration. *International Journal of Poultry Science*, v.5, p.360-364, 2006.

Oliveira, A.L.S.; Donzele, J.L.; Oliveira, R.F.M. et al., Exigência de lisina digestível para suínos machos castrados de alto potencial genético para deposição de carne magra na carcaça dos 15 aos 30 kg. *Revista Brasileira de Zootecnia*, v.35, n.6, p.2338-2343, 2006.

Oliveira, P.B.; Murakami, A.E.; Garcia, E.R. et al., Influência de fatores antinutricionais da leucena (*Leucaena leucocephala* e *Leucaena cunningan*) e do Feijão Guandu (*Cajanus cajan*) sobre o epitélio intestinal e o desempenho de frangos de corte. *Revista Brasileira de Zootecnia, Viçosa,* v. 29, p.1759-1769, 2000.

Oliveira Júnior, G.M. Relações triptofano e treonina digestíveis com lisina digestível em dietas para leitões pós-desmame criados em ambientes com e sem desafio sanitário. *Tese (Doutorado em Zootecnia),* 99f. UFV: Viçosa, 2012.

Oliveira, V.F.; Lopes, J.L.; Abreu, M.L.T. Treonina digestível em rações para matrizes suínas em lactação. Informativo Técnico Nº. 165 2014. Access: 20/07/2014. Avaiable: www.sossuinos.com.br/Tecnicos/ info165.htm.

Oliveira, W.P.; Oliveira, R.F.M.; Donzele, J.L. et al., Redução do nível de proteína bruta em rações de frangos de corte em ambiente de estresse por calor. *Revista Brasileira de Zootecnia*, v.39, n.5, p. 1092-1098, 2010.

Opapeju, F.O.; Krause, D.O.; Payne, R.L. et al., Effect of dietary protein level on growth performance, indicators of enteric health, and gastrointestinal microbial ecology of weaned pigs induced with postweaningcolibacillosis. *Journal of Animal Science,* v.87, p.2635-2643, 2009.

O'quinn, P.R.; KNABE, D.A.; WU, G. Arginine catabolism in lactating porcine mammary tissue. *Journal of Animal Science*, v.80, p.467–474, 2002.

Parsons, C.M.; Hashimoto, K.; Wedekind, K.J. et al., Soybean protein solubility in potassium hydroxide: an *in vitro* test of *in vivo* protein quality. *Journal Animal Science*, v.69, p.2918-2924, 1991.

Pereira, L.E.J.; Mello, H.V.; Leão, M.I. Farinha de vísceras de aves em substituição ao farelo de soja na alimentação de suínos em crescimento e terminação. *Revista Brasileira de Zootecnia*, v.23, n.6, p.930-939, 1994.

Pesti, G.M.; Bakalli, R.I.; Driver, J.P. et al., Comparison of Peanut Meal and Soybean Meal as Protein Supplements for Laying Hens. *Poultry Science,* v.82, p.1274–1280, 2003.

Pervin, S.; Singh, R.; Hernandez, E. et al., Nitric oxide in physiological concentrations targets the translational machinery to increase the proliferation of human breast cancer cells: involvement of mammalian target of rapamycin/ eIF4E pathway. *Cancer Research*, v.67, p.289–299, 2007.

Phelps, R.A. Cottonseed meal for poultry: From research to practical application. *World's Poultry Science Journal*, v.22, p.86-112, 1966.

Pimentel, A.C.S.; Dutra Júnior, W.M.; Ludke, M.C.M.M. Substituição do milho e do farelo de soja por sorgo e farelo de caroço de algodão extrusado em rações para frangos de corte. *Acta Scientiarum Animal Sciences*, v.29, p.135-141. 2007.

Prawirodigdo, S.; Batterham, E.S.; Andersen, L.M. Nitrogen retention in pigs given diets containing cottonseed meal or soyabean meal. *Animal Feed Science Technology*, v.67, p.205-211, 1997.

Remond, D.; Buffiere, C.; Godin, J.P. et al., Intestinal inflammation increases gastrointestinal threonine uptake and mucin synthesis in enterally fed minipigs. *Journal of Nutrition*, v.139, p.720-726, 2009.

Ringel, J.; Susenbeth, A. Lysine requirement for maintenance in growing pigs. *Livestock Science*, v.120, p.144–150, 2009.

Rodrigueiro, R.J.B.; Rostagno, H.S.; Albino, L.F. et al., Exigência de lisina para frangas na fase de 1 a 4 semanas de idade utilizando a técnica de abate comparativo e balanço de nitrogênio. . In: CONFERÊNCIA APINCO, 2008, Santos. Anais... p.113, 2008.

Rodrigues, P.B.; Rostagno, H.S.; Albino, L.F.T. Aminoacidos Digestíveis Verdadeiros do Milheto, do Milho e Subprodutos do Milho. *Revista Brasileira Zootecnia*, v.30, p.2046-2058, 2001.

Rossoni, M.C.; Donzele, J.L.; Oliveira, R.F.M. et al., Níveis de treonina digestível para suínos machos castrados, de alto potencial genético para deposição de carne, na fase de terminação. *Arquivo Brasileiro de Medicina Veterinária e Zootecnia*, v.60, n.4, p. 884-889, 2008.

Rossoni, M.C.; Donzele, J.L.; Silva, F.C.O. et al., Exigência de lisina digestível de fêmeas suínas selecionadas para deposição de carne magra, na carcaça dos 15 aos 30kg. *Revista Brasileira de Saúde e Produção Animal,* v.10, n.3, p.586-595, 2009.

Rostagno, H.S.; Jr, J.G.; Albino, L.F.T. et al., Níveis de glicina+serina em rações de pintos de corte. In: CONFERÊNCIA APINCO, 2003, Campinas-sp. Anais... p.105, 2003.

Rostagno, H.S.; Albino, L.F.T.; Donzele, J.L. et al., Tables for Poultry and Swine: Composition of Feedstuffs and Nutritional Requeriments, 3ed. Federal University of Viçosa, Viçosa, 252p., 2011.

Roth-Maier, D.A., Böhmer, B.M.; Roth, F.X. Effects of feeding canola meal and sweet lupin (*L. luteus, L. angustifolius*) in amino acid balanced diets on growth performance and carcass characteristics of growing-finishing pigs. *Animal Research*, v.54, p.21-34, 2004.

Roth, F.X.; Meindl, C.; Ettle, T. Evidence of a dietary selection for methionine by the piglet. *Journal Animal Science*, v.84, p.379–386, 2006.

Rutz, F. Proteínas: Digestão e Absorção. In: Fisiologia Aviária Aplicada a Frangos de Corte. MACARI, M.; FURLAN, R.L.; GONZÁLES, E.; editores.2ª ed. FUNEP, 2002.

Sá, L.M; Gomes, P.C.; Cecon, P.R. et al., Exigência nutricional de treonina digestível para galinhas poedeiras no período de 34 a 50 semanas de idade. *Revista Brasileira de Zootecnia*, v.36, n.6, p. 1846-1853, 2007.

Sá, L.; Nogueira, E.T. Atualização das relações valina e isoleucina com a lisina na proteína ideal para frangos de corte e suínos, 2009. Avaiable: <http://www.lisina.com.br/publicacoes_detalhes.aspx?id=2179>. Access: 14 julho 2014.

Salfen, B. E.; Acarroll, J.; Keisler, D.H. et al., Effects of exogenous ghrelin on feed intake. weight gain. behavior. and endocrine responses in weanling pigs. *Journal Animal Science*, v.82, p.1957–1966, 2004.

Santos, F.A.; Donzele, J.L.; Oliveira, R.F.M. et al., .Exigência de metionina + cistina digestíveis em suínos machos castrados de alto potencial genético na fase dos 60 aos 95 kg. *Revista Brasileira de Zootecnia,* v.36, p.2047-2053, 2007.

Santos, F.A.; Donzele, J.L.; Silva, F.C.O. et al., Níveis de lisina digestível para suínos machos castrados de alto potencial genético dos 95 aos 125 kg. *Revista Brasileira de Zootecnia*, v.40, n.5, p.1038-1044, 2011a.

Santos, F.A.; Donzele, J.L.; Silva, F.C.O. et al., Levels of digestible methionine+cystine in diets for high genetic potential barrows from 95 to 125 kg. *Revista Brasileira de Zootecnia*, v.40, n.3, p.581-586, 2011b.

Saraiva, E.P.; Oliveira, R.F.M.; Donzele, J.L. et al., Exigências de treonina digestível para leitoas mantidas em ambiente termoneutro dos 15 aos 30 kg. *Revista Brasileira de Zootecnia*, v.36, p.1861-1867, 2007a.

Saraiva, E.P.; Oliveira, R.F.M.; Donzele, J.L. et al., Exigências de treonina digestível para leitoas mantidas em ambiente termoneutro dos 30 aos 60 kg. *Revista Brasileira de Zootecnia*, v.36, p.1854-1860, 2007b.

Schöne, F.; Tischendorf, F.; Kirchheim, U. et al., Effect of high fat rapeseed press cake on growth, carcass, meat quality and body fat composition of leaner and fatter pig crossbreeds. *Animal Science*, v.74, p.285-297, 2002.

Shannon, M.C.; Allee, G.L. Protein and amino acid sources for swine diets. *Nutrition Guide*, p.01-07, 2005.

Shemin, D. & Rittenberg, D. The utilization of glycine for the synthesis of porfiryn. *Journal of Biological Chemistry*, v.159, p.567-568, 1945.

Silva, E.L.; Silva, J.H.V.; Filho, J.J. et al., Redução dos níveis protéicos e suplementação com metionina e lisina em rações para poedeiras leves. *Revista Brasileira de Zootecnia*, v.35, n.2, p.491-496, 2006.

Silva, E.P. Avaliação nutricional de farinhas de vísceras de aves e a utilização em rações de frangos de corte. Dissertação de Mestrado, Universidade Federal Rural de Pernambuco, Recife, 131p. 2009.

Summers, J.D.; Bedford, M.; Spratt, D. Amino Acid Supplementation of Canola Meal. *Canadian Journal of Animal Science*, v.69, p.469-475, 1989.

Sung, Y.J.; Hotchkiss, J.H.; Austic, R.H. et al., L-arginina-dependent production of reactive nitrogen intermediate by macrophages of an uricotelic species. *Journal of Leukocyte Biology*, v.50, n.1, p.49-56, 1991.

Suryawan, A.; Escobar, J.; Frank, J.W. et al., Developmental regulation of the activation of signaling components leading to translation initiation in skeletal muscle of neonatal pigs. *American Journal of Physiology*, v.291, p.E849–E859, 2006.

Tavernari, F.C.; Bernal, L.E.P.; Rostagno, H.S. et al., Relação metionina + cistina / lisina digestível para frangos de corte cobb. *Revista Ceres,* v.61, n.2, p.193-201, 2014.

Thacker, P.A.; Newkirk, R.W. Performance of growing-finishing pigs fed barley based diets containing toasted or non-toasted canola meal. *Canadian Journal Animal Science*, v.85, p.53-59, 2005.

Toledo, G.S.; López, J.; Costa, P.T. et al., Aplicação dos conceitos de proteína bruta e proteína ideal sobre o desempenho de frangos de corte machos e fêmeas criados no inverno. *Ciência Rural*, Santa Maria, v.34, n.6, p.1927-1931, 2004.

Trindade Neto, M.A.; Lima, J.A.F.; Fialho, E.T. et al., Farelo de glúten de milho (FMG) para suínos em crescimento e terminação (desempenho). *Revista Brasileira de Zootecnia,* v.24, p.108-116. 1995.

Tuitoek, K.; Young, L.G.; De Lange, C.F.M. et al., The Effect of Reducing Excess Dietary Amino Acids on Growing-Finishing Pig Performance: An Evaluation of the Ideal Protein Concept. *Journal Animal Science, v.*75, p.1575-1583, 1997.

United States Department Of Agriculture (USDA). Feed and Animal Management for Swine (Growing and Finishing Pigs). *Nutrient Management Technical Note* No.3, October. 2003.

Utiyama, C.E. Utilização de agentes antimicrobianos, probióticos, prebióticos e extratos vegetais como promotores de crescimento de leitões recém desmamados, 2006. Tese (Doutorado em Ciência Animal e Pastagens)- Escola Superior de Agricultura "Luiz de Queiroz", Universidade de São Paulo, Piracicaba, 2006.

Van Dijk, A.J.; Everts, H.; Nabuurs, M.J.A. et al., Growth performance of weanling pigs fed spray-dried animal plasma: a review. *Livestock Production Science*, v.68, p.263-274, 2001.

Waldroup, P.W. Cottonseed meal in poultry diets. *Feedstuffs,* v.53, p.21-24, 1981.

Waterhouse, H.N.; Scott, H.M. Effect of different proteins and protein levels on the glycine need of the chick fed purified diets. *Poultry Science,* v.40, p.1160-1165, 1961.

Wang, X.; Qiao, S.Y.; Yin, Y.L. et al., A deficiency or excess of dietary threonine reduces protein synthesis in jejunum and skeletal muscle of young pigs. *Journal Nutrition*, v.137, p.1442–1446, 2007.

Wang, W.; Zeng, X.; Mao, X. et al., Optimal Dietary True Ileal Digestible Threonine for Supporting the Mucosal Barrier in Small Intestine of Weanling Pigs. *Journal of Nutrition*, v.140, p.981–986, 2010.

Worsae, H.; Schmidt, M. Plasma cortisol and behaviour in early weaned piglets. *ActaVeterinaria Scandinavica,* v.21, p.640–657, 1980.

Wu, G. Papeis importantes da glutamina na nutrição e produção animal. In: AminoGut. Ciência e prática na nutrição de leitões, 2008.

Wu, G.; Bazer, F.W.; Davis, T. A. et al., Important roles for the arginine family of amino acids in swine nutrition and production. *Livestock Science,* v.112, p.8–22, 2007.

Wu, G.; Fang, Y.Z.; Yang, S. et al., Glutathione metabolism and its implications for health. *Journal of Nutrition*, v.134, p.489–492, 2004.

Zanella, I.; D'ávila, A.; Raber, M. Proteína ideal: conceito e aplicação na nutrição de aves e suínos. Anais... ZOOTEC 2004, 28 a 31 de maio de 2004 – Brasília, DF.

Zanotto, D.L.; Ludke, J.V.; Guidoni, A.L. et al., Utilization of canola meal in diets of growing and finishing pigs. *Archivos de Zootecnia*, v.58, p. 717-728, 2009.

Zardo, A.O.; De Lima, A.J.M.M. Alimentos para suínos. Boletim informativo BIPERS. Centro Nacional de Pesquisa de Aves e Suínos (EMBRAPA) e Associação Riograndense de Empreendimento de Assistência Técnica e Extensão Rural (EMATER/RS), 1999. Available in:

http://file.aviculturaindustrial.com.br/Material/Tecnico/alimentosuino.pdf. Access: 15/07/2014.

Zhang, H.; Yin, J.; Li, D. et al., Tryptophan enhances ghrelin expression and secretion associated with increased food intake and weight gain in weanling pigs. *Domestic Animal Endocrinology*, v.33, p.47–61, 2007.

Zhang, Z.F; Kim, I.H. Effects of dietary threonine: lysine ratios on growth performance, blood urea nitrogen, and nitrogen balance in weaned pigs. *Journal of Applied Animal Research*, DOI: 10.1080/09712119.2013.875915, 2014.

Zhang, G.J.; Xie, C.Y.; Thacker, P.A. et al., Estimation of the ideal ratio of standardized ileal digestible threonine to lysine for growing pigs (22–50 kg) fed low crude protein diets supplemented with crystalline amino acids. *Animal Feed Science and Technology*, v.180, p.83–91, 2013.

INDEX

A

B

C

D

H

I

J

K

L

M

N

O

P

Q

R

S

T

U

V

W

X

Y

Z